Contents

Part IV. The Tools of Positive Family Therapy

Part V. Conflict Contents and Conflict Dynamics

Part VI. The Five Steps in Positive Family Therapy and How They Operate

List of Stories

A Story for the Positive Process: The Dream

A Middle East king had a frightening dream. He dreamt that all his teeth fell out, one after the other. Very upset about this, he summoned his dream interpreter. The man listened with great concern to the king's account of his dream and said to him, "Your Majesty, I have bad news for you. Just as you lost all your teeth, you will lose all of your family, one after the other." This sad interpretation kindled the king's rage. The dream interpreter, who had nothing better to say, was thrown in jail at the king's command. Then the king summoned a different dream interpreter. This one heard him tell the dream and then said, "Your Majesty, I have good news for you. You will become older than all of your family. You will outlive them all." The king rejoiced and rewarded the man richly for saying this. But the courtiers were very surprised. "Your words were really no different from your poor predecessor's. But why was he punished, while you received a reward?" they asked. The lucky dream interpreter replied, "You are right. We both interpreted the dream in the same way. But it is not a question of what you say, but also how you say it."

Six Theses of Positive Family Therapy

1. Self-Help: Positive Family Therapy proceeds from the word *positum,* i.e., from what is factual and given. Disorders and conflicts within a family are not the only things that are factual and given. The family also brings with it the capacity for dealing with the conflicts. In the framework of Positive Family Therapy, the patient relinquishes his role as patient and becomes the therapist for himself and his environment.

2. Universal charater: Positive Family Therapy views an illness as more than a mere feature of the individual person. It is also a reflection of the quality of the relationships within the family and society. Positive Family Therapy offers a basic concept for approaching all illnesses and disorders.

3. Transcultural Aspect: Transcultural thought is the basis for Positive Family Therapy. This holds true for the person as a member of a group and as an individual. Every person stands within the cultural sphere he grew up in. But he also has his own personal sphere as a result of his upbringing. This can lead to transcultural problems in dealing with his fellowmen.

4. Content aspect: Positive Family Therapy tries to answer the question "What do all people have in common, and in what ways are thcy different?" To answer this, the therapy describes an inventory of conflict contents. Within the individual, these are as powerful as in the family and society. The conflict contents are the basis for the therapeutic instruments used in Positive Family Therapy.

5. Metatheoretic aspect: Since Positive Family Therapy proceeds from the contents, it offers a concept within which various methods and directions can be used to supplement each other.

6. Relativity of family ties: Positive Family Therapy is a special form of therapeutic thought. Although the family stands in

the center, the therapy does not limit itself to the family as the therapeutic unit. Rather, it tries to look at the family members as individuals and include social factors in the treatment.

If we transfer the ideas of Positive Family Therapy to the entire realm of social relationships (groups, peoples, nations, and cultural circles), we can perhaps develop a social theory that, alongside economic factors, would focus on the formational possibilities of concrete interpersonal relationships.

Introduction

If two people each have an apple and then exchange them, they still have only one apple.

But if the same two each have an idea and exchange them, each thereby has two ideas.

—after George Bernard Shaw

When people in Europe or the United States meet aquaintances on the street, they say hello and then begin a game where the question "How are you?" automatically elicts the reply "Fine. And you?" In the Mideast, the dialogue runs a bit differently, for the people there are more likely to ask, "How are you? And how is the family?" Asking about the family is an accepted part of the ritual. Rarely does a person fail to include it when starting up a conversation.

Behind these differences in the rituals, there seem to be different concepts of what constitutes identity. In the West, the ego is the center of the individual's identity. It is assumed that if I am okay, then things are also fine with my family, my job, et cetera. In the Mideast, however, there is a different point of reference. A person there would reason "If my family is well, then I am fine, too." The family is an integral part of one's identity and sense of worth.

When the Massai of Kenya meet, they greet each other with the following words: "I hope your cattle are well!" Cattle are their only source of livelihood, and so they devote much trouble and care to looking after them. Their cattle provide them with their three staple foods: milk, meat, and blood.

The concepts described here have their advantages and disadvantages: close ties with the family and the breaking of these ties. It is not my concern here to prove that one concept is better than the other. My aim is simply to consider the conditions in which such concepts develop, to describe their consequences, and to look for ways of utilizing them in the context of therapy and self-help.

TRANSCULTURAL ASPECTS OF THE POSITIVE FAMILY THERAPY

Since 1968 I have been working on a new method of psychohygienics and psychotherapy. I have tried to examine the behavior and conflicts of patients from viewpoints that were somewhat unconventional. The motivation for starting this new method may have been that I am, personally, in a transcultural situation.

It is the effect of a new development that national, ethnic, and cultural groups open themselves to the outer world, i.e., toward other groups. This trend carries new possibilities, which we shall describe as transcultural problems. They can therefore be reduced to two basic problems:

1. What is it that all men have in common?
2. By what do they differ?

An essential characteristic of the group is the standards valid in a group, which are reproduced for the individual as psychosocial standards with emotional components. There are, for instance, different attitudes, expectations, and behaviors regarding the psychosocial standard "politeness" in two different cultures (e.g., the Federal Republic of Germany and Iran). Typical representatives of both groups place great importance on "politeness." Lack of politeness can lead to social, psychic, and psychosomatic disturbances in both groups. However, each understands something different by "politeness."

In Germany when you are invited to a meal, it is considered polite to eat all the food that you are offered. It is considered old-fashioned to leave some food for the sake of politeness. If you finish all the food that is offered, it is considered a compliment to the hostess.

A German visitor to Iran became sick. She complained:

> *I don't want to look at any more food. The first week that I was here I was invited to the houses of different families nearly every day. My hosts were very kind and did everything to pamper me. But the amount of food became too much for me. When I had finished my portion—and it was always very good—they would fill my plate again. Not wanting to be impolite, I would finish that, too. But they would continue to give me more, and this continued until I almost vomited. Consequently, in sheer self-defense I had to abandon all consideration for my hosts and leave the food. Still, my conscience bothered me because they had been so kind and nice.*

This visitor would not have felt guilty if she had known what she finally learned—leaving some food on her plate is considered polite in Iran.

This does not mean that one model is better than the other, but that they complement each other with regard to the totality of human experience. The transcultural aspect provides a more extensive alternative interpretation. According to the cultural and historical evaluation, an illness or a symptom can be given different significance.

From these aspects, my attention was drawn to the meaning of social standards for the socialization as well as for the development of interhuman and intrapsychic conflicts, and I found in Oriental as well as in European and American patients that behind the existing symptoms, as a rule, were conflicts the origins of which are usually found in a number of recurring behavior standards.

These experiences and reflections prompted me—in the field of psychotherapy as well—to regard the individual not merely in isolation, but also in the context of his interpersonal relationships and—as was the case in my own development—his "transcultural" situation, the things that in fact make him what he is. The transcultural approach colors the whole of Positive Psychotherapy. Part of my work involves investigating the relationships between culture and disease and between cultural concepts in twenty different cultural groups.

THE POSITIVE CONCEPTION OF MAN

Medical, psychological, and psychiatric terms are not used without regard for what is involved. They must be understood in terms of the theories and scientific concepts that created them, and they are part of the history of these theories. A term used in connection with its theory acquires a meaning that presupposes knowledge of the theoretical premises involved, as well as the possible diagnoses and therapeutic measures. In order to understand the word *superego* it is necessary to be familiar with at least the basic principles of psychoanalysis. To understand the meaning of *support* in psychotherapy, some knowledge of the theory of learning and its application in behavioral therapy is required.

Positive psychotherapy, dealing as it does with basic human abilities—potential and realized—is in a position to get through to people from different social backgrounds and to shed light on transcultural problems. The principles of education, therapy, and psychotherapy have always been derived from the conception of man prevailing at any given time. This conception is formed by the experience gained with parents and peers and by those beliefs that have been assimilated from others or that are part of tradition. They are group-specific and in the broadest sense dependent on the system of values associated with the philosophy of life and religion prevalent at any particular time. An important reason for my own concern with Positive Psychotherapy may also have been that I am in a transcultural situation. I am an Iranian, but have been living in Europe since 1954. In this time, I have noticed that many modes of behavior, habits, and attitudes are evaluated completely differently in the two cultural groups. This observation, which I had already made during my childhood in Teheran, applies particularly to prejudices of a religious nature. As Baha'i, we were always in the cross fire between our Islamic, Christian, and Jewish schoolfellows and teachers. This led me to reflect on the relations existing between the religions and on interpersonal relationships. I came to know the families of my schoolfellows and to understand their behavior on the basis of their philosophy and their conception of the family. Later I witnessed similar confrontations, when during my specialist training I experienced the tension existing among psychiatrists, neurologists, and psychotherapists or psychoanalysts and the violence with which psychiatric and psychoanalytical ideas conflicted. I began to take an interest in the intrinsic nature of this type of tension and the reason behind it. Of particular importance for me was the realization that the family could have another form and organization from those I had experienced in my childhood and youth. The family in which I grew up comprised not only my parents and brothers and sisters, but a multitude of relatives and other dependents with whom we had close ties. In it I experienced a feeling of belonging to a group, of reciprocal care and security, but also a feeling of dependence and restriction. The typical American family, which sets great store by its independence, seemed to me—with all its advantages—to complement the Oriental system. I came to regard the family as a kind of switchboard where certain capabilities and human possibilities are developed and others are suppressed. The family thus exerts a powerful influence in many areas of life. It helps to determine one's choice of a career and spouse and affects how one relates to other people and faces one's own future.

These ideas led me to look at people primarily in terms of their interpersonal relationships. Even in psychotherapy, I no longer regarded a patient as an isolated individual. As in my own development, I began to look at a person's transcultural situation. I wanted to find out what shapes him into what he is.

This transcultural view is evident throughout all of Positive Family Therapy. We give it such great importance because it helps us understand the individual's conflicts. It can also be important in dealing with such social issues as the treatment of illegal aliens and refugees, foreign aid for the Third World countries, problems in dealing with members of other cultural systems, interracial and transcultural marriages, prejudices, and alternative life-styles adopted from other societies. It can also be applied to political problems brought about by transcultural situations.

This book would have been impossible without the family I grew up in and the one I call "my family." I am especially grateful to my wife, Manije, and sons, Hamid and Nawid, whose probing questions continually motivate me to reassess my own ideas. Special thanks also go to my colleague Dieter Schoen for his helpful suggestions. I also thank Hans Deidenbach, a behavioral therapist, and Willi Koehler, who read the manuscript and offered many suggestions. My spiritual teachers, Mr. A. Furutan, Mr. A. Faizi, and Dr. D. Ruhe, provided the impetus for work and contributed much help along the way. My secretaries, Mrs. Krieger and Mrs. Hofmann, have given invaluable help through their untiring and meticulous work. I would like to express my warm thanks to the translator, Mrs. Martha Rohlfing, of Chicago.

Of special importance to me was the creative atmosphere within the Psychotherapeutic Discovery Group in Wiesbaden (PEW) and the German Association for Positive Psychotherpy (DGPP). The participants in these groups provided an excellent example of how members of various therapeutic disciplines, social workers and practitioners can work together meaningfully and positively on a day-to-day basis.

Wiesbaden, September 1985 Nossrat Peseschkian, M.D.

Part I

Introduction to the Theory of Positive Family Therapy

It is not possible to fly with one wing alone! Should a man try to fly with the wing of religion alone he would quickly fall into the quagmire of superstition, whilst on the other hand, with the wing of science alone he would also make no progress, but fall into the despairing slough of materialism.

—Abdu'l Bahá, Paris talk

THE PROPER PRAYER

While on a trip, Abdu'l 'Bahá, the son of Bahá'u'lláh, the founder of the Bah'i religion, had been invited to dinner with a family. The wife had good intentions and wanted to show her great culinary artistry. When she brought out the food, she apologized for the fact that it was burnt. While cooking it, she had been reading prayers in the hope that the meal would be especially successful. Abdu'l 'Bahá answered with a friendly smile and "It's good that you pray. But next time you're in the kitchen, pray from a cookbook."

This story illustrates the close ties between religion and daily life, which the devout adherent of a religion clearly perceives. It deals with the difference between religious and everyday tasks and aptly points out religious narrowmindedness and the mental disorders that stem from the confrontation with ecclesiastical rules of morality.

1. THE SITUATION IN SCIENCE, RELIGION, EDUCATION, AND PSYCHOTHERAPY

The current situation of psychotherapy needs the development of methods that are at the same time economical and effective. Positive Psychotherapy (Differentiation Analysis) is a method of that kind. It works as a therapy concentrating upon conflict.

Our present-day situation is interpreted and explained in different ways. People talk of the age of fear, the age of depression, the age of aggression, the age of the loss of trust, and the age of hopelessness. When we look more closely, we realize that complaints and symptoms are being used as a basis for these interpretations. Behind these symptoms we can discover certain one-sided views, one of which seems to play a central role.

The scientific aspect is overemphasized and the religious is neglected, or the religious aspect is overemphasized and the scientific neglected. The neglected area is usually pushed aside and frequently becomes the source of conflicts and difficulties.

The present situation in science, religion, education, and psychotherapy is in many respects similar to the following Oriental story:

> *An elephant was being exhibited at night in a dark room. People crowded around to look at it. Since it was dark, the visitors could not see the elephant so they tried to touch it to get an idea of what it looked like. But as the elephant was very large, each visitor could only touch a part of the animal and describe it the way he had felt it. One of the visitors, who had touched the elephant's trunk, said that the elephant was like a thick column. Another, who had touched the elephant's tusk, described the animal as something pointed. A third, who had touched an ear, said the elephant was like a fan. And the fourth, who had stroked the*

back of the elephant, insisted that the elephant was straight and flat as a bed.

—After Mowlana, Persian poet

RELIGION AND PSYCHOTHERAPY

To transfer this example to science, religion, education, and psychotherapy: everybody sees correctly, but not everybody sees everything. Thus it is not surprising that so many parents, pedagogues, and therapists are at a loss when they realize this lack of unity.

When we look back into history, we see that in earlier times science and religion were considered as one. As the area of work was divided more, religion and science also diverged. This differentiation not only brings opportunities, it also causes limitations. Just as science brought forth a series of schools of thought (often in intense rivalry with each other), there are also different directions in religion. However, just as the scientific schools complement one another, religions can also work together. An essential part of the conflicts goes back to the fact that the aspect of development and the dimension of time are not taken into consideration. What is religion? What is psychology?

Religions give us norms that govern interpersonal relationships and the position of man in the world picture. Thus religion is concerned with giving meaning. Psychology considers questions concerning the conditions of these norms that can be scientifically comprehended, the conflicts that arise from different norms, and the possibilities that the individual has to work them out. Thus the task of psychology is to describe the meaning. For instance, religions tell us that we should not tell lies. Psychology asks why someone lies; why another, when people lie to him, cannot trust anyone anymore; why someone boastfully portrays himself as more than he is; why another presents himself to others as being less than he is.

Religion itself is partly a topic of psychology. However, it is not so much religion itself that is put to the test but rather the behavior and attitudes of the individual believer or the group of the religious community. Why does someone become rigid, dogmatic, and develop prejudices in the area of religion? Why do others want to discard everything religious in content and form? Why do people today tend to put taboos on religion, perhaps more than they used to do with sexuality? Why does someone tend to oscillate between the single religious interpretations and not be able to identify with a religion? The connection between religion and psychology becomes more distinct when we consider man's possibilities for development.

Man develops by acquiring a relationship with himself, his parents, a partner, his children, his fellowmen, his profession, and finally a religion. Every human being develops in these areas in some form. These forms belong to the reality of our lives, and they have functional coherence.

This means that when someone has difficulties in one area, for instance at work, this difficulty can be transferred to the partner or the church; it can influence his relationship with his fellowmen and finally can lead to his placing no value on religion at all.

2. WHAT IS "FAMILY THERAPY"?

Be ye as the fingers of one hand.
—Bahá 'u' lláh, *Hidden Words*

Looking at recent publications, one has the impression that family therapy is a new concoction from the psychotherapist's alchemic kitchen. It is met with diverse reactions. Some regard it suspiciously, seeing it as a deviation from traditional therapeutic methods; others praise it as an important advance in the treatment of psychoses. Still others view it as a special method for dealing with children.

The conventional view of family therapy is a narrow one. According to this view, therapy treats an entire group—at least father, mother, and child—not just an individual patient. In the therapeutic situation, these family members present a major component of their everyday life.

But this kind of process has only limited application. It cannot be carried out, for instance, if the original family no longer exists, if members of the family are unwilling to start therapy, or if the tensions in the family are so great that it is impossible to gather the group under one therapeutic roof.

This is why we try not to look at family therapy simply as a particular therapeutic arrangement. Instead, we interpret it as a special way of thinking, one that does justice to man's social nature.

When we speak of family therapy, we mean a method of treatment that encompasses a range of possibilities, from individual treatment at one end of the scale to ecotherapy at the other. But regardless of where the therapy is situated between these two poles, it focuses on the family and on the conditions existing within it.

3. WHAT DOES "POSITIVE FAMILY THERAPY" MEAN?

Know ye not why we created you all from the same dust? That no one should exalt himself over the other?
—Bah'u'lláh, *Hidden Words*

Traditional psychotherapy derives its image of man from psychopathology. It therefore deals with illnesses. The goal of the treatment is the elimination of these illnesses, much like the surgical removal of an unhealthy organ. Sometimes, of course, the illness is actually eliminated, but this does not necessarily mean that health is restored.

The first thing a patient learns in therapy is that he can get the therapist's attention only by virtue of his illness. As a result, the disorder moves more and more into the foreground, thereby limiting the number of therapeutic remedies available.

This imbalance is historically and culturally determined. It is an imbalance we could minimize if we were willing to consider other ways of thinking—ways that offer different interpretations of the illnesses and suggest alternative strategies for treatment.

Symptomatic procedures and traditional therapy can deal with the child only after he has fallen into the well—in other words, after the damage has been done. A preventive (family) therapy, on the other hand, must of necessity be a "positive" family therapy. It doesn't just look at the areas where there is a disorder; it also considers the capabilities that exist in the individual and in the family. In its original meaning the word *positive* (Latin *positum*) refers to the factual, the given. The "givens" are not necessarily conflicts and disorders, but can also be the capabilities that each person carries within him. In therapy we are interested primarily in man's capacity for self-help and his ability to deal with conflict.

In order to understand observed behavior, we need background information that will give us the criteria for making judgments later on. This means we must examine both the transcultural conditions and the personal circumstances that give meaning to the individual's behavior. We emphasize the significance of the psychosocial background against which the specific conflict dynamic develops. We then try to broaden our concepts of the illnesses and supplement them in terms of new therapeutic possibilities. In taking a positive approach, we try to develop an overview that will encompass as many interpretations as possible. It is our goal to influence the family's understanding of itself and the illness. In this way, we can control the disturbing influence emanating from areas outside the realm of medicine.

The transcultural view begins with the realization that the relationship to an ailing person varies from culture to culture. There are also differences in how one faces the suffering and evaluates the illness subjectively. Furthermore, the family and the group—regardless of the cultural setting—can react to the patient in different ways.

If we look at the historical development of the ideas surrounding illness, we see that the views prevailing in our society today are not as obvious and inevitable as they seem at first glance. The development of these attitudes (cf. Peseschkian, *Positive Psychotherapie* [Frankfurt: 1977, S. Fischer]) reflects the nature of the association with the sick person and, consequently, the ways his family can deal with him.

The individual concept of illness includes the ideas held by a particular person. They can be understood only by examining his personal development and the system of relationships within his family.

This relativization of the concept of illness is especially important for the dynamics within the family. It gives the illness a definite function and sets the tone for the relationships between family members. This is the case regardless of whether the illness is pyschic, psychosomatic, psychotic, or somatic.

We investigate how the same disorder or illness is perceived and assessed in other cultures, how the people in a particular culture or family face the illness, what particular meaning the conflicts have for the individual, and which contents they address.

Let's take the case of a daughter who can't get along with her mother and wants to leave home. As an expression of the crisis affecting both parties, we find typical generation conflicts, separation anxieties, aggressions, and guilt feelings. We can relativize these reactions by asking ourselves how the mother and daughter would face this situation in a different culture, such as the Mideast. We can then proceed to investigate how other people in the same culture—perhaps again a mother and daughter—would have dealt with this problem in a different epoch. Finally, we look at what this separation process means for the daughter and the mother. At this point, we also determine which contents are involved (thrift, order, sexuality, trust, hope, promptness, et cetera), which functions the conflict has in the development of family ties, and what positive aspects it transmits for the people involved.

This process brings the neurotic one-way communication to a halt and gives both mother and daughter new insights into their relationship. They can then choose from a number of alternatives to see which might solve their problem.

4. Guidelines for the Reader

If you give someone a fish, you feed him only once.
If you teach him how to fish, he can feed himself forever.

—Oriental wisdom

The first part of this book defines the family from the transcultural point of view and explains previous methods and approaches to family therapy. In giving this information, we will dispense with the narrower views of family therapy and try to present it as a method of therapeutic thought.

The second part deals with the tools of Positive Family Therapy. These tools form the basis for the therapeutic work:

The positive process means that every person has a number of capabilities at his disposal; each disorder and illness carries out a definite function for the patient and his social environment. In other words, they contain positive aspects. From symptoms we then move on to the conflict.

The four ways of dealing with conflict enable us to gain access to the previously held ideas about the illness. If we study the one-sided ways people try to handle their conflicts, we can interpret them as limited ways of dealing with reality. This interpretation gives us a model that can help us control and broaden the person's range of reactions to reality.

The four model-dimensions are related to the history of the patient's family and serve as a map for our journey into the past.

The basic capabilities form the potential inherent in every individual, regardless of his physical and mental health and his social situation. They are the basis for human relationships and represent areas that all people have in common, irrespective of individual and cultural differences.

The actual capabilities are the psychosocial norms transmitted by the family. They provide the family members with the rules that govern their interaction. In family therapy, these norms are

identified by using the Differentiation Analytical Inventory (DAI). It reflects the contents behind personal, family, and social conflicts.
The three stages of interaction are a model for interpersonal problems. In terms of content, these problems are shaped by the basic capabilities and the actual capabilities.
The five-stage Positive Family Therapy is a therapeutic strategy in which family therapy and self-help are intertwined. As we lead the family step by step toward self-help, our motto is "If you need a helping hand, look for it at the end of your own arm."

"Part 3: The Practice of Positive Family Therapy" deals primarily with the concepts that represent, in terms of contents, an advancement of the views of the actual capabilities. They are the "helmsmen" that intervene in the lives of everyone. In this section of the book, case histories illustrate how the concepts determine the development of the conflict and the ways it can be handled. The case histories also show how Positive Therapy can be conducted. From the dynamics of the concepts we developed a "family tree" of the concept, thus offering the possibility of a therapy that can span several generations. The final part of this chapter deals with transcultural concepts. Since these concepts permit insight into the dynamics of how conflicts develop, this final section can stimulate the reader to experiment with alternative modes of thought.

The process set forth in this book is patterned after the method I have introduced in my other books. *Positive Psychotherapie* (1977), *Psychotherapie des Alltagslebens* (1977), and *Der Kaufmann und der Papagei* (1979). All these books have been published by the S. Fischer Company

Since the theoretical formulations of my work are given extensive treatment in my book *Positive Psychotherapie,* we have not made them the focus of this book. Instead, we assembled the instruments of Positive Psychotherapy and then tried to apply them to the particular concerns of family therapy. We tried to extend those ideas of Positive Psychotherapy that deal with the psychological relationships within families. This goes along with my belief that any form of treatment loses out on significant possibilities if it fails to look at the family background, either directly or indirectly.

Equally important is my interest in Oriental stories as resources and communication aids, as instruments in my field of specialization, psychotherapy. An additional factor has been the connection between the wisdom and intuitive thoughts of the Mideast and the new psychotherapeutic methods of the West.

Part II.

Transcultural Psychotherapy (The East-West Concept)

Every age has its own problem and every soul its particular aspiration.

—Bahà'u'llah

1. Social Changes and the Image of Man

A ROOFTOP GARDEN AND TWO WORLDS

One summer night, the members of a family slept in the garden on top of their house. To her great displeasure, the mother saw that her son and his wife (whom she barely tolerated anyway) were snuggled up against each other. Unable to bear this sight, she woke them both up and cried, "How can you sleep so close together in this heat? It's unhealthy and dangerous." In another corner of the garden, there slept her daughter and son-in-law, whom she adored. They were sleeping apart from each other, with at least a foot of space between them. The mother woke them up gently by saying, "My darlings, how can you sleep so far apart when it's as chilly as this? Why don't you warm each other up?" The daughter-in-law heard this. She sat up and, with a loud voice, uttered the following words like a prayer: "How mighty is our God. A rooftop garden and such a variable climate."

In the past fifty years, social conditions have changed by leaps and bounds. To be sure, human consciousness perceives these changes only to a limited degree. People cling to outmoded ideas and thus retain an antiquated idea of the human race. If you compare the social conditions today with those of earlier times, you are struck by one particular development, which can be described through the following four processes:

a) *Population growth:* At the time of Christ, there were about 200 million people living on earth. By 1950 it was 3 billion. It is estimated that world population will be 7 billion at the end of this century, 12 billion in the year 2030, 24 billion in 2070, et cetera (Niemöller, 1968).

This process involves more than a quantitative increase, for it is closely connected to a number of problems that will grow in importance—problems such as how to feed all these people, how to deal with pollution, and how to control the socioeconomic forces.

We must keep in mind that the slope for population growth is considerably higher than the slope for increases in output. This prognosis means that in the year 1999, the percentage of undernourished peoples will rise from 57 to 75 afflicting a total of 5.6 billion people. In other words, for every person who has enough to eat, there will be three others with insufficient diets (Niemöller, 1968). Quantitative change thus ushers in a restructuring of society.

b) Urbanization: The process of urbanization is an indirect result of the population explosion and depends to a large extent on the conditions for production. An agrarian society, for example, needs land for agricultural production. The organization of cities, on the other hand, relies more on manual and industrial forms of production. Until a few generations ago, most of the world's people were rural, but the onset of industrialization triggered a migration to the cities. This trend can be seen in almost all parts of the world—at different rates, of course. The consequences of urbanization threaten to grow to unforeseen dimensions and will certainly produce acute problems for child rearing and interpersonal relationships. Advances in hygiene, for example, have already become widespread, but they often produce a sterile lifestyle. The child who played around on the manure pile in an agrarian society is now more likely to be confined to an apartment in the modern city. This limited environment diminishes his opportunities for development and stirs up new conflicts. In many cases, the pathway to the playground exists only in theory or is an even worse alternative. The spatial density of the city offers the individual a more intense relationship with his social environment. The number of contacts is quite high, of course, but one's ability to deal with them remains limited. In earlier times, the members of the grand family provided the environment for education; today the neighbors fill this role—sometimes with unhappy consequences for everyone. The mother of a nine-year-old child once complained, "I'm having trouble with my neighbors on account of my son. They keep telling me I should watch after him more closely and discipline him more. It bothers me when other people want to butt in. They complain that my little boy has no business being out on the street. But he knew I've given him permission. They don't like him because he doesn't do as they say. If someone finds some litter in their yard, they blame it on him. These problems with the neighbors are really getting me down. I cried the whole afternoon because of how unfair they are to my boy."

c) Differentiation and specialization: Scientific progress in conjunction with social and economic developments has led to a process of differentiation. In some ways, this concept overlaps with that of the division of labor. In former times, one person could have a number of roles, like chief, priest, judge, and physician. Today we find the various functions separated and so specialized that many occupations are defined by a limited number of specific operations carried out by the laborer. Workers on an assembly line are a good illustration of this.

Increased differentiation has produced new occupational forms, careers, social roles, branches of science, and administrative agencies.

Analogous processes of differentiation have taken place within the family. Functions that the grandparents used to fulfill are now divided up over many social organizations. Today a child is born in a hospital and is looked after by a nurse. The child's upbringing is then carried out by the father, mother, grandparents, babysitters, kindergarten, school, summer camp, day-care center, et cetera. These divisions within the child's upbringing produce problems that must be faced in his formal education. Our times have thus created conditions that influence human development even if we prefer to close our eyes to them.

d) Integration: As a result of all these developments, national, ethnic, and cultural groups are beginning to open up to the outside world, i.e., to other groups. A trend of this kind is accompanied by new possibilities, new *transcultural problems.* Here is an example. In 1978 there were some 90,000 Turks living in West Berlin. Although this is a relatively closed group, one that is trying to hold on to its religious and cultural identity, there are a number of points of contact between the group and the other people of Berlin. This leads to conflicts about norms and values and produces compromise on both sides. The result is a transcultural exchange that transcends cultural, national, and philosophic lines. The most impressive models for this exchange are the transcultural marriages where the parties involved come from widely diverse cultural backgrounds. Aside from learning to iron out their personal differences, they have to come to terms with the particularities of their historical and cultural origins. This problem can be seen in all its nuances, as when a tourist or foreign worker comes to a new land or when the nationals encounter this "intruder." Similar problems occur on economic, social, and political levels. A good example of this is the exportation of technology to the so-called developing countries. The introduction of these sophisticated methods of production creates far-reaching changes in those societies. Family units that had been very strong—such as had existed in the Mideast—are torn apart. Further changes take place in the relationships between family members, in the family's defense systems, and in the family's opportunities to be together.

> These changes become obvious when we take as an example the differences between a typical Mideast bazaar and a department store in the Western world. In the bazaar, economic gain is not the sole motivating force; the rituals of bargaining and the accompanying interpersonal contacts play a significant part in the life of the tradesman. In a large department store, however, the functions of buying and selling are clearly separated, thus removing much of the need for personal contact. These economic developments affect religions and philosophical ideas as well as daily life. Conservative religious groups tend to view these changes with suspicion. They fear that the changes will destroy their own displays of power, perhaps even their autonomy as a group.

The social changes brought about by population growth, urbanization, differentiation, and integration have produced a development that Toynbee refers to as the destruction of values. As a matter of fact, there are today almost no firmly held relational systems for such things as "the right education." In earlier times, religion and morality supplied the criteria, standards, and goals for education and social behavior. They showed what was right or wrong, good or bad. Today social groups and institutions have evolved into the transmitters of our social norms. Instead of the destruction of values, we find a displacement of values in the sense of a change in function. An example of this is when people neglect their personal relationships because of the demands of their own need for achievement.This is a conflict that characterizes the relationship between the Mideast and the West. Another example can be found in sexual morality, whereby the concept of fidelity has undergone a reevaluation.

Changes in the environment do not occur without having an impact on society and the people living in it. Role expectations placed on the individual by society and by himself change in accordance with the conditions and needs of that society. Bahá'u'llah put it in these words: "Every age has its own problem and every soul its particular aspiration."

The changes taking place in the world today no longer permit a family to act as if it were a closed group that needed to heed only its own rules. From the closed world view of earlier times, a new, more open world has emerged. It is no longer simply a question of reaching the unimpaired structures and relational forms within a family. Pluralistic coexistence in many families and groups—each espousing diverse philosophical, ethical, and religious systems and living according to particular methods of production and rules of conduct—is becoming the standard for the educational task within the individual family. This makes the transcultural point of view a foundation for interpersonal relationships. It can be found throughout all of Positive Family Therapy.

Examples for Medical Expressions and Some Views of Illness

Behavior/ Concept	*West*	*East*
Illness	When a person is sick, he'd like to have rest. He is visited by few people. Visits are also perceived as social control.	Here, when a person gets sick, the bed is installed in the living room, e.g., by a footstool. The sick person is the center of attention and is visited by many family members, relatives and friends. For visitors to stay away would be seen as an affront and lack of sympathy.
Separation Anxiety	Expectations and transmissions are mostly directed towards individuals or small groups. For example, only a limited number of guests are invited. One is disappointed when someone backs out or doesn't show up. "Why couldn't he come over? Isn't it good enough for him here?" "If he's so unreliable, we can't invite him any more."	The simple transmission is replaced by multiple transmission, which also provides a socially recognized insurance against separation anxiety. One not only invites guests, whose nonappearance means a great disappointment, but rather makes many people his guests. If someone comes late or stays away, the presence of the others guarantees the success of the evening.
Anxiety	Modern psychotherapy likewise knows these three kinds of basic anxieties.	Oriental philosophers distinguish three types of anxieties, which they call

	Fear of the past and fear of the present are called historically experienced anxieties, and fear of the future, as existential anxiety. Prayer and meditation as measures against fear of the future have stood the test of time for centuries, and work as means of imparting trust and hope. This only becomes problematical if the requirement of prayer suppresses the active provision for the future.	basic anxieties: fear of the past—cause: injustices; treatment: pardon and forgiveness. Fear of the present—expressed through loneliness; treatment: withdrawal from the social environment and asceticism. Fear of the future—expressed through a feeling of lack of meaning and goals; treatment: prayer.
Leisure Time	"When my husband comes home, the food has to be ready. Then he sits down in front of the TV and drinks his beer, then goes to bed and reads his newspaper!"	"My husband relaxes best when he chats with guests. Therefore, my main job is to serve the guests in the evening."
Narcissism	"I've worked for you all day, and insist that for your part you have consideration for me and accept my rules of the game." This interpretation is narcissistically based. The one who in the family demands consideration and an undisturbed evening at the same time requires recognition by the family of his achievement.	"I have reached the point where I can entertain you all, I have provided for you all through my work and efficiency in business." The oriental concept illustrates an extroverted narcissism. The father is not content with his narrow family circle, but rather needs a big forum for his narcissistic desires.
Ego Strength	The expression belongs to the liberal willpower model of bourgeois society, in	The basis of identification is not the I, but rather the We. I can only be well if I

	which social compensations and fantasy take a back seat to the overcoming of reality as justified by the achievement motive. For psychoanalysis, ego strength and ego maturity are central concepts.	live in harmony with my social environment.
Solidarity	Self reliance and autonomy are held to be desirable. Children leave home early: "I'm old enough and can stand on my own two feet!" "You're old enough now and must know what you do." Being too close to the parental family is experienced as a threat to self reliance.	Great stress on family solidarity. Parents often send their children several thousand kilometers away to study and know that through the "social umbilical cord" and through contact, letters, etc., the dependence on the parents and the family ties persists in spite of the distance.
Solitude	"The strong are most powerful alone." The ability to be selfreliant, independent and alone is seen as a strength. No one finds anything amiss if someone goes for a walk alone and loses himself in thought.	The search for solitude and withdrawal from current social events are seen as a disturbance of trust. Mistrust arises: What's happening with him? Is he offended? We can surely help if he is griefstricken.
Consideration	Loud behavior is seen as impolite, disobedient and inconsiderate. "As children, we were only allowed to talk when we were asked." "Playing is forbidden during the midday rest!" "Don't be so loud, you surely know that the neighbors complain!"	It is held to be normal if one is loud, especially if the children are loud. Less consideration is given to the neighbors, who also in general are not disturbed by the noise of children.

Pain	The sufferer mostly stands alone, either because he wants to "solve his own problem" or because the others have no time for him or say: "Let him see how well he gets along." In addition, the sufferer often has to bear the feelings of indifference, rejection or sadism.	The sufferer—whether suffering from material need or psychological and physical pain—is taken into the social body of the extended family and cared for. The responsibility is borne collectively. This involvement gives the one affected a certain emotional security.
Alcohol	Alcohol can be called the drug of the masses. In this sense, alcohol is an illness of the peoples and is spread over practically the whole world. Indulgence in alcohol has a long and rich tradition. Alcohol, like most other intoxicants, has a sacred significance. It is a generally recognized "polite" custom to dring alcohol on determined occasions. This ranges from the diplomatic reception to passing around the mug after passing an exam. Since drinking alcohol forms a part of it, it is hard for a teetotaller to avoid this "duty." He easily becomes an outsider, and is considered impolite. A French wine grower is integrated into his society in spite of his consumption of alcohol. Neither he nor his milieu would find his behavior abnormal.	Moses made no commandment or prohibition concerning alcohol. Nor in the Gospel of Jesus Christ do we find any express prohibition. In accordance with the sense of the Christian message, however, moderation is necessary in all areas of life. Islam has a severe prohibition of alcohol. Even moderate indulgence in alcohol threatens a person's esteem. The Bahá'í Faith forbids indulgence in alcohol, except in the case of a medical prescription. "Experience has shown how much abstinence from tobacco, wine and opium brings health, strength, spiritual happiness, a sharp power of judgement and vital physical energy."

Drugs	A person who is dependent on drugs quickly falls into the behavioral pattern of a marginal man, and perhaps of a criminal. The social ostracism is bound to affect him if he has no physical pain that might justify the use of drugs. Here the limits of what is tolerated are very narrow, because of the perception of grave dangers facing society because of drugs.	Here one encounters people who in spite of lifelong use of drugs have remained respected members of their society, and who show no major damage either physically or mentally. The smoking of hashish in place of the forbidden alcohol is also widespread, causing perhaps even greater damage and likewise contradicting the will of the Prophet, although perhaps not expressly. But here too it may be observed that the regular use of drugs is predominantly restricted to circles on the margin of society.
Schizophrenia	With the internment in a clinic, the reference persons, who previously had cared for the patient, seem to give up their duty to provide care and their readiness to work together with the institution. A relationship with the patient which still existed at the beginning often wanes in the course of the stay at the clinic. The patient falls into increasing isolation, making his rehabilitation more difficult. The patient often seeks causes for his illness in events in his environment, e.g., imagining that	Here, the patient is kept as long as possible in the family. Often the extended family even resists the expulsion of a sick member of the family. The milieu shows great concern, and offers help through visits, presents, etc. Latent in this is the danger that this folk therapy may not be very objective, and may be emotionally depressive, confining and anxietyproducing in its effects on the patient. Here, the patient often perceives that the cause of his illness is a hex which has been put on him by neigh-

	he is being disturbed by police radar. Such manifestations on the part of the patient are to be seen as pathological, and at the same time lead to a distancing from his environment.	bors or relatives. Such an imagination seems to be plausible within the oriental thought world, and assures to the affected person strengthened emotional support together with an impressive therapy. The reputation of being possessed can thrust a previously unknown person into the limelight of public attention, giving him considerable influence for a while.
Depression	Middle Europeans and North Americans develop depressive moods because they lack contact, they are isolated and suffer from a paucity of emotional warmth. The contents of the depressions differ in many respects from one another. In the foreground are anxieties which can be related to external appearance, beauty and sexual potency, but also to social isolation, orderliness, cleanliness, and especially thrift.	In the orient, depressions are more likely to develop because people feel overburdened by the narrowness of their social obligations and involvements, which they cannot back out of. In terms of contents, anxieties about fertility, social appearance and the relation to the future are in the foreground.

Transcultural problems—that is, those problems that develop in the clash between various models of culturally determined values and behavior—are just one particular kind of conflict. As a problem of communication, this conflict illustrates the various concepts and their problematic entanglement. As has already been pointed out, the members of various cultural groups adopt typical features that affect their interpersonal re-

lationships and expectations as well as their outer appearance. In the same way, the individual brings with him his own "educational sphere." Out of it are developed the various systems of relationships and value structures that in turn structure people's understanding of each other. But they can also provoke conflicts between individuals and within the individual himself. In other words, every person is a tiny but nevertheless semiopen system with his own tradition linked up in some way to the traditions of his social environment. The prototype for these "microcultures" is the family.

2. Practical Aspects of the East-West Concept in Family Therapy

ABOUT THE COURAGE TO RISK A TEST

A king put his court to a test for an important post. Powerful and wise men stood around him in great numbers. "You wise men," said the king, "I have a problem, and I want to see who of you is in a position to solve it." He led the men to a huge door, bigger than anyone had ever seen. The king explained, "Here you see the biggest and heaviest door in my kingdom. Who among you can open it?" Some of the courtiers just shook their heads. Others, who were counted among the wise men, looked at the door more closely but admitted they couldn't do it. When the wise men had said this, the rest of the court agreed that this problem was too hard to solve. Only one vizier went up to the door. He checked it with his eyes and fingers, tried many ways to move it, and finally pulled on it with a hefty tug. And the door opened. It had just been left ajar, not completely shut, and nothing more had been needed but the willingness to realize it and the courage to act boldly. The king spoke: "You will get the position at the court, for you don't rely just on what you see or hear; you put your own powers into action and risk a test."

TRANSCULTURAL PSYCHOTHERAPY

Today the transcultural problem is increasing in importance. In earlier times, people were separated by great distances and came into contact with each other only in unusual circumstances. Today, however, modern technology has dramatically increased the probability of transcultural contact. Just by opening up the morning paper we step beyond the limits of our daily lives and establish contact with the problems faced by other people from varying cultural circles and groups. As a rule, we understand these events only to the extent that we are used to them from our own way of thinking. We easily tend to criticize, laugh at other people, or damn them for their alleged backwardness, naieveté, brutality, or incomprehensible lack of concerns.

But our contact with foreign cultures is not simply transmitted by the media, but takes place on a real plane. Illegal aliens might live in our community, and at work we perhaps stand right next to a member of another culture. When we go on vacation, we are attracted to the differences we find in foreign cultures and lands that we visit. To be sure, these contacts don't always take place without trouble. Generally there are all sorts of misunderstandings, fears, aggressions, mistrust, and prejudices that can mushroom into hatred toward a particular group.

Transcultural psychology deals with the causes and prerequisities for these disorders in human interaction. In my experience, I have found that a particular situation has developed in which transcultural problems are partially expressed clearly and openly, but also partly sublimated and finely differentiated under the surface of daily interaction. I am speaking here of the marriage between people of two different cultures.

The transcultural world of work, alongside the private sphere and transcultural politics, is growing in importance, regardless of whether foreign workers find employment in a country or if the country "exports" such laborers. Based on the foreseen developments, one can anticipate that transcultural problems will pose one of the major challenges for the future.

In the transcultural process, we are concerned with the concepts, norms, values, behavioral styles, interests, and perspectives that are valid in a given culture. Such an approach encompasses the characteristic traits of a population. It uses the collective norms and behavioral patterns as a guideline. One attempt to objectivize these values is comparing the laws and legal norms of a nation. But even more interesting for me, more stratified and more dazzling, are the day-to-day behavioral patterns, conflicts, and possible solutions that are typical for a culture—that is, they can be observed again and again and are very regular. But it is precisely here that there is a two-fold danger for the transcultural process: First, the transcultural starting point tries to mediate between the various views, to find forms of metacommunication in discussions about the conflicts and thereby break down the prejudices. On the other hand, the type casting associated with the crosscultural process—labels like "the German," "the Persian," "the Middle Easterner," "the Italian," "the Frenchman," et cetera—can lead to stereotypes and prejudices. For these reasons it seems important to remember that transcultural descriptions are types—abstractions and statistical majority relationships—which always allow exceptions and can be reputed by the individual case. In this sense, paradoxes are possible, and we encounter these paradoxes frequently. The "Prussian" Middle Easterner who takes punctuality, orderliness, and exactness so very seriously is just as common as the "Middle Eastern" Prussian, who would be particularly suited for a Middle East bazaar because of his tolerant and lax attitudes about punctuality. Another difficulty becomes apparent: What is this thing called culture, which is the subject of this transcultural question? Does there still exist a closed, mature, clearly delineated cultural unity?

Cultural units can be drawn on a map. This shows that they are connected in some way to interpersonal life, to the geographical prerequisities of a landscape, to the common history and the socioeconomic level that has been achieved. Within a unit that is conceived of in this way, there are subgroups that are distinguished from other groups by virtue of their customs or overlap with the life-style of another cultural circle. This latter development can be seen in many forms today as the confrontation between the traditional agrarian social forms and the industrial society. These confrontations are taking place most acutely in Third World countries and in the Middle East.

Social systems, forms of production, and philosophies intermingle with cultural distinctions. A method of looking at crosscultural phenomena is thus insufficient if it only considers the large, transmitted cultures. It must also look at subcultures groups, living communities, and the family. And just as every culture has its special norms and values, so each of these subgroups enjoys its own characteristics, right down to the family itself, where, for example, there are concepts that can be understood only by the family members and that contain norms that may or may not agree with those of the dominant social order: "At our house, it wasn't important whether you came late. The main thing was that you were there. I've always found that very pleasant. For me it was always a sign of trust and love whenever my family welcomed me openly even if I was late. This period when I was free of the pressures to be prompt was a paradise for me, but it didn't last once I had to start going to school. There was continuous quarreling about that, and it is still going on" (42–year–old wife of a patient with heart trouble).

Just as there are cultural circles, there are also educational circles where each person develops this own cultural system and confronts other systems with it. The principle underlying the

transcultural problem thus becomes the principle for interpersonal relationships and the mental processes for dealing with conflict. In this way, it becomes a subject of psychotherapy.

The goal of such therapy must not be to renounce cultural, group, familial, and personal distinctions. Rather, what seems important is the realization of individual characteristics as well as cultural uniqueness, when there exist on the other side possibilities for dealing with conflicts that may arise. To use an example from linguistics: it is important that each person keep his own language, but he should be able to speak a language that will enable him to make himself understood to other people. Transcultural psychotherapy tries to achieve such a language as metacommunication, as communication about conflicts.

THE "STRANGE" PARTNER: "MY HUSBAND IS A SADIST"

The German wife of an Iranian doctor complained about her husband, "My husband is a sadist. He's too rough with our child. He squeezes him like you'd squeeze a lemon, pinches him, bites him on the arm, and slaps him on the back and stomach. I have some understanding of affection, but that isn't affection anymore, but brutality and sadism. I am afraid my husband will raise our boy to be a masochist who enjoys being tormented. He treats me the same way, and I have to admit that he simply repulses me."

What should be done in such a case? One can take the woman's comments seriously. Her descriptions do indeed point to sadistic elements. Taken as is, biting, hitting, and pinching are all attributes of torment, and here it appears to be something that is fun for the husband. As a sadist, he would then be the sick one and would have to be treated accordinly. But it is not certain at this point whether he is ready or willing to take on the patient role and let his behavior he called into question. But if we should change our position in judging this case and proceed from the common expectations of a Middle European, the problem of the "sadist" appears in a different light.

In the Middle East, children are frequently hugged and kissed. The kiss as the epitome of love and care is often linked to a slight biting, while hugging is linked with a bit of pinching of the hips or breasts. The child might feel some discomfort with this painful expression of affection, but this is diminished by the other person, usually the father, laughing out loud, designating the whole situation as "good" and "pleasant." The child thus does not react by crying, as would probably be the case if the person had done something improper. The child adopts the father's laughter and, for his part, experiences the whole situation, including the pain, as a sign of connectedness, affection, and emotional security.

In the Middle East, mutual touching and hugging take place throughout the person's entire life. Friends and acquaintances are often embraced on the street, kissed, and pinched teasingly. Middle Eastern men usually develop similar rituals of intimacy with their wives. But sometimes it happens that the wife, the partner, does not understand these gestures as expressions of tenderness.

This can especially be the case with Western women who are not familiar with this special tenderness in their own development and interpret it consequently as "crudeness," "brutality," and "sadism."

Different Tenderness

Many Europeans find it hard to get used to the rituals of tenderness in the Middle East, since it goes somewhat contrary to the contact limitations they learned in the course of their socialization. On the other hand, people from the Middle East find it hard to act in a European way—distanced—in a European setting and to suppress spontaneous reactional patterns that were common practice in their home culture. Hugging is replaced by handshaking or merely nodding. Tenderness is suppressed and hidden behind more matter-of-fact forms of contact.

It is almost a model case for a Middle Eastern man to marry a European woman and adopt to Western behavioral norms during his residency in Europe. But he starts having trouble the moment he returns to his homeland with his wife. The behavioral norms that he couldn't develop in Europe are now required of him at home. He embraces his friends and acquaintances, kisses them, and acts in the ways he was used to acting as a child. For his European wife, this can all become a bitter disappointment: The emphasis on family relationships, the pronounced contact rituals, and the emphatic openness in her husband's homeland are strange to her. She doesn't feel she belongs. Almost automatically the alternative takes shape: who does my husband love more—me or his family and friends? In the European cultural areas, especially in Germany, physical contact seems less desired. In infancy, of course, physical tenderness receives a lot of attention, but in the following years it is replaced more and more by expectations of achievement and is shifted to the verbal area. From late childhood on, tenderness is regarded as "childish." A "grown-up" is someone who can do what is expected of him without intimacy and without emotional dependencies. Touching is often experienced as an intrusion into one's personal freedom and is thus something one does only to a limited extent.

In place of physical communication we find verbal forms of contact: people fulfill the function of embracing or even friendly pinching by paying compliments, using irony, witty conversation, jokes, and suggestive or obliging comments.

Who Is Sick?

Against this background, the behavior of the "sadistic husband" takes on a different meaning. It is less a personal "sick" deviation; rather, it becomes meaningful within the given cultural framework.

The experiment in rethinking that we just posed has special meaning for the treatment. Earlier, the husband seemed disturbed and sick; his behavior ran counter to the "valid" behavioral norms. But new the problem becomes a question of interpersonal, even transcultural matters. Typical expectations and behavioral patterns of the Middle East and the West meet in the ideas of a German physician and her husband.

The doctor had brought her complaints to my office with the unconscious motive of finding in the therapist someone who would ally with her against her husband. In the treatment, which was conducted as family therapy, the husband outlined how he had acquired his behavior. In so doing, he was repeatedly astonished by the connections that now became apparent to him. "I have always experienced on my own person the things I was taught. But that my education and upbringing still influence my behavior now is something I hadn't been aware of until now."

The wife, however, was not receptive to becoming aware of her strong dislike of any powerful physical contact. In her parents' authoritarian home, where the emphasis was on ambition, achievement, and neatness, she associated her urge to touch with her fear that her father would beat her. In their house there was very little hugging, people remained at a distance from each other, and physical contact was reduced to shaking hands and other mild forms of contact, such as "laying your arm on someone's shoulder" or "touching someone on the cheek." For her, the behavior of her husband was thus aggressive and injurious.

The following concepts were crystalized:

Husband's concept: Hugging someone closely, biting, and pinching are proper ways to express love and affection.

Wife's concept: Vigorous hugging, biting, and pinching are aggressive, injurious, and sadistic. The proper ways to express love and affection are caressing and gentle hugging.

For both of them, the wife as well as the husband, there began a period of relearning and differentiation. The treatment lasted ten sessions spread out over half a year. The instruments of Positive Family Therapy were put into use. The main themes that become focal points were the relationship to the body (tenderness) and the actual capabilities for punctuality, orderliness, achievement, and contact. Both partners, and also their child, brought their personal difficulties and their typical transcultural problems into the process. The therapeutic emphasis was on the wife during the stages of observation/distancing, inventory, and situational encouragement. For the husband, it was the stages of inventory and verbalization. For the son, it was mainly observation/distancing and verbalization. The family members together, as a family group task, were to work through the stage of goal expansion. Here the problems of attachment came to the foreground and the positive aspects of independence for the family members were singled out.

The doctor's wife, who had called her husband a sadist, withdrawn from him emotionally, and developed signs of aversion to sex, reported, "I have learned to know my husband as a completely new man. Previously, a lot of things about him were unusual and weird to me. My dislike for him had increased in the past few years, mainly becaus he was raising our son in ways I found repulsive. But now that I know why my husband reacted that way and, more important, why I was so against it emotionally, I get along a lot better with him. For me it was a real step forward when I was finally able to tell my husband what kind of physical pleasure I wanted from him. I've completely loosened up, I must say. When I'm really feeling bold I even give him a teasing little slap on the fanny."

"COMPANY COSTS TOO MUCH MONEY"

A thirty–year–old German woman described how it was when her husband would get home from work: "When he comes home, supper has to be ready. Then he sits down in front of the T.V., has a beer, then goes to bed and reads the paper. His motto for these hours of the day is 'I want my peace and quiet.' And he never budges from this."

In contrast to this, a Persian woman told me, "My main task is to take care of our guests in the evening. My husband relaxes best when he is chatting with guests. . . ."

So we can see that there are no hard-and-fast rules about how to relax. You relax the way you have learned how to.

The German husband of a patient once told me, "I'm bored to death in the evening. But I have no better idea of what to do, so I just sit and watch T.V."

But the wife had the chance to do something about their long-neglected social contacts and invited some company over. Here the husband could learn to relax in an entirely new way.

But there were problems in this, which, however, could be easily solved. The husband sought contact, but avoided it at the same time, because having people over involved expense. The wife was afraid that company would mess up the house, and for this reason she was satisfied to spend the evenings quietly at home. But eventually the alternative for relaxation was tried, and this expanded and enriched the lives of both marriage partners.

Each of these interpretations contains some narcissism. The one who demands consideration from his family and an undisturbed evening at home also wants his family to acknowledge his accomplishments: "I've worked all day for you and want something in return. I want you to be considerate and accept my game rules."

On the other hand, the Middle East concept represents an extroverted narcissism. The father is not satisfied just with his small family circle, but needs a larger forum for his narcissistic desires: "I've achieved enough to be able to entertain all of you; through my work and good business sense I have seen to all of your needs."

Both these views represent extreme concepts between which a number of variational forms are possible. None of these concepts is inherently conflict-laden. Indeed, each concept is justified within the corresponding cultural situation.

We don't just have one or two concepts at our disposal. Each of us also has individual nuances of these concepts. For example, as long as the wife is willing to adopt for herself a withdrawal from contact and to associate social contact with achievement (visits from business friends et cetera) the situation may remain relatively free of conflict. But if the partners have different concepts or one person adheres to differing concepts, there is a higher chance of conflict: "You can work as hard as you want. But I don't want to sit through a boring business meal. I want my own circle of friends and my own freedom." Or "For a long time I was able to identify with the existing demands for accomplishment, but I suffer again and again from the fact that I am isolated and, because of my work, have few friends and personal acquaintances." Or "The content of my life is careful, exact, and conscientious work. To accomplish that, I have to have a quiet evening and go to bed early. Visiting with guests would be a waste of time."

SEPARATION ANXIETY also takes on a new meaning against the transcultural background. In the West, separation anxiety is often intensified by the fact that expectations and transferences are usually directed toward individual persons or small groups. You invite a small group of guests, usually weeks in advance, in writing if possible, and express an occasional fear about your expectations: "What will our guests think of us?" "We hope they'll enjoy it here," et cetera.

Strict game rules are operating here: One guest too many is almost as catastrophic as one guest too few. In the first case, the planning of the occasion is thwarted; in the second case, there are a lot of uncomfortable feelings and fears of separation: "Why didn't he come to our house? What did he want to achieve by that?" You tend to cover your hurt feelings by acting aggressively: "If someone is going to be that unreliable, we won't invite him again."

In the Middle East, there are other ways to prevent these kinds of anxieties. Not only do you invite a lot of people whose failure to come would be a disappointment to you, but you also invite a lot of people as your guests. The host's flexibility, his willingness and ability to provide lavishly, is an important source of satisfaction for him, and gives him stature in the eyes of his guests. The simple transference is dissolved by multiple transference. This represents at the same time a socially acceptable way of insuring against separation anxieties.

But this attitude presupposed "sacrifice." You must be ready to put up with the disarray that the guests can produce in the house. You have to be willing to spend money, since there is expense involved with having guests. This, of course, is made easier to endure by virtue of the solidarity created by your other guests. If a guest comes late or doesn't show up at all, the others make up for it; you don't end up spending the evening alone; the evening is a social success anyway, and the host is less obligated to entertain one individual guest during the evening. The guests can mingle and entertain each other, and the host functions more as a catalyst. He makes introductions, mentions the guests' particular interests, initiates conversations, offers food and drink, and lets his guests react to each other spontaneously. In so doing, he receives a lot of direct and indirect social recognition. He's what one would call the "emotional leader" in group psychology, and he is less vulnerable to the frustrations that come from hour-long conversations and fruitless attempts to make contact with someone: "Last week we invited two colleagues. They couldn't talk about anything but their work. As human beings we didn't get a bit closer than we were before. The evening was such an effort for me that I am not interested in ever inviting them over again."

Separation anxiety is dealt with according to the sociocultural situation and takes on a different meaning because of it. Object loss acquires its psychic meaning in a similar way. It is not derived solely from an infantile problem, but is determined in content by sociocultural norms. A partner is considered irreplaceable, but the minute he is unfaithful, he is rejected. A guest who repeatedly arrives late is rejected in Western circles because he is considered too unreliable. One doesn't want to have anything to do with him, even though there are a lot of interests in common. Dynamic concepts like narcissism, separation anxiety, object loss, regression, et cetera are thus made more precise in terms of their contents. Along with the characterizing epignetic susceptibilities for conflict and the structures of experience, there comes the content aspect by which sociopyshcological, social, and cultural factors are brought into the psychotherapy. We start with these transcultural considerations and the idea that the various individual concepts correspond in many respects to the various transcultural concepts. This enables us to interpret illnesses and disorders in various ways: Let us first take the organic illnesses—for example, a carcinoma. This illness has a narrowly defined organic condition and, based on previous experience, an extremely unfavorable prognosis. Yet we see that people who have this illness react to their situation in different ways and place their illness in different value systems.

We see patients who resist their illness in a desperate manner, gain no insight into the "meaninglessness" of their illness, or expect their death passively and with resignation. On the other hand, we find patients who actually are able to comfort their doctors and attendants, keep active, and help people around them to deal with their own fears of death. This is all in spite of or because of their suffering.

In other words, depending on the various concepts, even the most serious illnesses acquire different subjective meaning and

can influence the subjective feeling of well-being and experiencing of pleasure. One sees this most pronounced in psychic and psychosomatic disorders where the experiential aspect is also in the foreground in an etiological sense.

FAMILY: SECURITY OR NARROWNESS

In new psychotherapy, there is a tendency to emphasize the independence of the patients and thus to support their detachment from their family home: "You must finally separate from your parents." This means something should be done to counteract the infantile, childish dependencies that often enough determine a person's behavior. But one shouldn't make a golden rule out of this recommendation, for the significance of the family ties can vary, regardless of whether they are real or exist only in the perceptions of the person concerned. A spacial separation from parents and other close figures still says nothing about whether a person has removed himself from them emotionally as well. In reverse, one can live with another person and still acquire independence, maturity, and autonomy. The ability to detach oneself is affected by various factors: for one thing, by one's life story; for another, by the viewpoint of various cultural circles.

In the Orient, the choice of a spouse is strongly directed by the relatives and the larger family. In a transference sense, the family is a filter through which the aspirant must pass before he can even become a serious candidate for the marriage. There are selectional criteria that such a candidate must fulfill: Does he come from a good family? What is his profession? Is he independent? The reverse applies to the woman: Is she from a good family [however one interprets this idea]? Is she a good housewife? Does she have a good reputation? These early decisions are made by the parents, aunts, uncles, et cetera. Then they present the candidate in an appealing way: "I have a good wife for you"; "She's from a good family"; "When the people have company, you can imagine how fantastically they have a party." In this way the marriage is prepared and determined in agreement with the family. The new marriage stands in a continuum with family tradition. In Central Europe, this tradition has a relatively minor meaning. It is a sign of independence and maturity to choose a partner on one's own initiative and with one's own criteria. The family's desires can pass almost as unconscious motives. But they can also be neglected in a demonstrative way: "I 'm not a child anymore and don't have to have my parents tell me whom I can marry." The criteria for selection are derived from the subjective interests of the individual: to have a caring or a self-reliant partner, to marry for money, or the generational duty to take a man or woman who will fulfill one's wishes. This selection process also effects one's relationship with the in-laws. A result of the independent selection of a partner is that the in-laws and the son-in-law or daughter-in-law must first get used to each other. The in-laws find themselves facing almost a *fait accompli* that they can either adjust to or more or less openly oppose. Since there is usually considerable spacial distance—moving in with the parents is not a good idea—one can usually avoid points of friction. But problems develop when the in-laws interfere in the couple's problems and exert moral pressure on their son or daughter to take sides.

In the Orient, the conflict with in-laws runs a different course. Here the parents, often more so than the people directly involved, set the ground rules for the choice of spouse. They thus were able to select a daughter-in-law or son-in-law who came closest to meeting their expectations. If one disregards the cases of a miscalculation, the conflicts generally develop from the close relationship between the married children and their parents. These relationships persist even after the marriage has taken place. In Europe the attention and excessive interference from the in-laws often arouse obvious suspicion or obvious jealousy. But in Iran these impulses are usually hidden behind the traditionally prescribed positive relationships to the in-laws. Even if there is some jealousy and rivalry, the Iranian wife knows that she is lost without an alliance with her mother-in-law, since such an alliance is born out of necessity. The mother-in-law problem is carried out under this omen under the cover of an emphatic "politeness."

But if open fighting begins, usually a mother-son alliance is formed, which is circumscribed by the saying "The elephant remembers India." The son remembers his obligations to his parents and thereby puts himself in conflict with his wife. In reverse, a mother will hardly over attack her son from behind. In her eyes, his faults are even virtues. She can forgive him as long as he just meets his obligations to her and the family. The daughter-in-law is thereby given some "consolation: "You should be satisfied. You have such nice kids, your husband is very generous, and you always have a lot of company. It's just not that important."

A LARGE FAMILY OR SOCIAL INSURANCE

In the Orient, people take a very uncomplicated attitude toward the future. In Europe, people make careful plans for at least the immediate future, money is divided up according to priorities, and Saving, as in Saving Money, is written with a capital S. But in Iran people like to spend their money on their children and their guests. Almost two-thirds of the earnings of a middle-class breadwinner goes for the children's education and for entertaining. It's almost impossible to save money, and quite often parents are without income in their old age and have to rely on what they invested in their children. Even socializing is a way of building up your reserves. Through unconditional investments for entertaining, you obligate yourself to other people, and they can then step in and lend a hand when things are not going so well for you. The mutual willingness to be of help works astonishingly well. A businessman can be helped in a bankruptcy; a father can be helped if money is tight. If the family provider dies, the larger family or clan will usually step in and take over the responsibilities of caring for his dependents. Even in the case of psychic problems, with depression, conflicts, and the helplessness of the elderly, the group, which also makes a lot of demands, now feels responsible. The person who is suffering is incorporated into the social body of the family and is taken care of. This solidarity also takes place after divorces, after the death of a loved one, during a marital separation, and even when the lovers are having a few problems. Responsibility is shared collectively. The family collective has a role that is similar to the social welfare policies in Europe. By making investments, obligations are created, and these are finally dissolved when a crisis occurs. But this form of action goes beyond the purely financial aspect. It also creates a certain sense of emotional security. Often, however, the persons involved and, to an even greater extent, people from other cultures perceive this as a kind of meddling.

It has been seen again and again that none of these cultural systems is inherently good. Their quality is proven by how they influence the people who live in them and by how much their game rules allow a constructive confrontation with other sociocultural systems. So there is much remaining that the people of various cultural systems could learn from each other—if only they would learn to understand each other.

Part III:

From Family Therapy to Positive Familiy Therapy

THE PROPHET AND THE LONG SPOONS

An orthodox believer came to the prophet Elijah. He was motivated by the question of hell and heaven, for naturally he wanted to live his life accordingly. "Where is hell—where is heaven?" As he said these words, he approached the prophet, but Elijah did not answer him. Elijah took the man by the hand and led him through the dark alleys into a palace. They passed through an iron portal and entered a large room crowded with many people, rich and poor, some huddled in rags, some adorned with jewels. In the middle of the room, a big pot of soup, called "asch," stood over an open fire. The simmering casserole spread a wonderful aroma throughout the room. Around the pot, crowds of hollow-cheeked and empty-eyed people jockeyed to get their share of the soup. The man who came along with Elijah was amazed when he saw the spoons the people carried, for the spoons were as big as the people themselves. Each spoon consisted of an iron bowl, white but from the heat of the soup, and way at the end, a small wooden handle. The hungry people greadily poked around in the pot. Although each wanted his share, no one got it. It was hard to lift the heavy spoon out of the pot, and, since the spoon was very long, even the strongest men could not get it in their mouths. The more impertinent people even burned their arms and faces or spilled the soup on their neighbors. Scolding one another, they fought and hit each other with the spoons they should have been using to quiet their hunger. The prophet Elijah took his escort by the arm and said, "That is hell' " They left the room and soon were no longer able to hear the infernal cries behind them. After a long journey through dark passages, they entered a different room. Here, too, there were many people sitting around. In the middle of the room there was again a pot of hot soup. Each of the persons there had a gigantic spoon in his hand, just like the ones Elijah and the man had seen in hell. But here the people were well nourished. Only a quiet, satisfied humming could be heard along with the sounds of the spoons being dipped into the soup. There were always two people working together. One dipped the spoon in the pot and fed his partner. If the spoon became too heavy for one person, two others helped with their implements to that everyone was able to eat in peace. As soon as one person had had enough to eat, it was another one's turn. The prophet Elijah said to his escort. "That is heaven!"

This story, which has been a part of oral tradition for thousands of years, is an accurate picture of life. It represents the things we see when we look at the problems within individual families—quarrels between parents, fighting among children, and the battles between parents and their offspring. We see it again in the way the individual confronts his surroundings and even in the disagreements between groups and peoples. The "hell" in the story exists when people work against each other or simply next to each other. "Heaven," on the other hand, comes about through the willingness to establish positive relationships. Both sets of people—those in heaven as well as in hell—have the same kinds of problems. How they solve those problems determines whether their life is heaven or hell.

Every family contains a bit of both worlds. The choice is up to us. Our chances of actually achieving the one we have chosen depend in large part on two things: first, our own experiences and how we have learned to solve problems, and second, our willingness to use that experience and share it with the people around us.

1. The Family as Hell

Happy families are all alike; every unhappy family is unhappy in its own way.

—Tolstoi, *Anna Karenina*

It is estimated 37 percent of the adults in West Germany are heavy drinkers. Of the 1.5 million who have drinking problems, some 10 percent of them are adolescents. In the last ten years, the number of alcoholics who have lost their jobs has tripled (Schaefer, 1978). Ten years ago, the ratio of female alcoholics to male alcoholics was one to ten. Today 31 percent of the people dependent on alcohol are women. In 1978 the people of West Germany spent 37 billion German marks for alcohol (*Medical Tribune,* Nr. 5, 1978). These statistics become important for family therapy when we consider the following ideas: Alcohol is a drug that produces a feeling of warmth, security, and comfort. It thus takes on many of the functions traditionally attributed to the family. In addition, alcohol is frequently an attempted form of self-medication, a way to solve one's problems (Battegay et al., 1979). The statistics on suicide—the second most common cause of death—are the most conspicuous indicators of the lack of emotional props within an affluent society, a welfare state. In West Germany, 14,000 people take their own lives every year, approximately the same number as are killed in traffic accidents. Along with these 14,000 suicides, there are 200,000 attempted suicides and, undoubtedly, countless others that go unreported.

At the first European police conference on youth, held at Aachen in 1977, the following data were made public: Between 1963 and 1976, the number of people suspected of crime rose 77 percent in the eighteen–to–twenty-one age group, 104 percent among minors, and 132 percent among adolescents. In most cases, these crimes involve vandalism and use of force. A third of the twenty-five–year–old men in Germany have been convicted of a misdemeanor or felony. Professor Kurt Nitsch, president of the German Association for the Protection of Children, spoke on the occasion of World Health Day in 1977 and noted that 25 percent of all children show serious behavioral disorders and that every third child feels lonely, neglected, and unhappy. The number of children killed by their parents is ten times as large as the number killed by sexual criminals. Estimates on child abuse have reached such high figures that this crime can now be considered the most common one.

Many people today sneer when they hear someone say that the family is a place of emotional security. These people are more likely to view the family as a place for suppression, misunderstanding, mutual irritation, narrow-mindedness, coldness, and isolation. They are the ones who would say, "I'm happy when I'm out of the house, when I don't have to face my folks, and when I can spend my time as I please." In this connection, Scharmann (1958) talks about defunctionalization, expressed most conspicuously in the decreasing role that the home plays in family life. In Scharmann's words: "The home is being stripped of its function as a place for work, interaction and relaxation. It is becoming a kind of loading dock, a gas station where members of the family show up only to eat and sleep" (cf. Rudorff, 1955).

The natural division of the family into generations leads to conflicts between the generations. These conflicts stem from the fact that members of the younger generation, at their particular state of development, have some trouble getting along with their parents, and vice versa. Either the young people try to distance themselves from their parents or they remain bound by confusions that are accompanied by ambivalent feelings. If the children then go ahead and renounce the family, they sense that something is missing and try to find a substitute for it. A nineteen-year-old student, for instance, entered psychotherapy because she was depressed. She brought members of her commune along to the sessions, explaining that "I won't have anything to do with my family anymore, but at least I have friends I'm comfortable with."

For children and adolescents, suicide and attempted suicide are particular ways of reacting to conflicts both within and outside the family. In this age group, we find two overlapping motives for suicide. The first of these is the child's feelings of being unwanted and superfluous of being a disturbing factor in the home. The emotional foundations of the family are disturbed. Interpersonal relationships are cold and impersonal. The parents either merely live alongside one another or find themselves involved in constant quarrels. Often the child is told that he is unwanted. His parents make it clear to him that his very existence disrupts their lives. Children and young people commit suicide so their parents will feel free to get a divorce. Sometimes the child thinks he can save the marriage and the family by sacrificing his own life. This attitude takes on new importance when we remember that the number of divorces is rising steadily.

But there is another motive that is even more common. At first glance, the families of child suicides or attempted suicides seem very normal. They are typical families where the parents appear to give their children a lot of attention and importance. The parents inspire in the children a desire for achievement, but this desire is often accompanied by the fear of failure. The child begins to feel that all his positive ties with the parents depend on his accomplishments. He fears he will be accepted only as long as he does well. This attitude doesn't even need to be verbalized within the family. It is conveyed so clearly through day-to-day activities that the child is able to say to himself, *At the dinner table my father looks at me very seriously. At that minute I know that the hour has come. He then comes out with the question "How was school today?," and I know I'm in for it if I didn't have a good day at school.* These correlations between achievement, self-esteem, family roles, and recognition from the family sometimes prevent the child from accepting poor grades, less than perfect accomplishments, and other shortcomings. At the moment, he finds it easier to simply end his life than to disappoint his parents or receive this disapproval. These kinds of attitudes within the family are based on outside values to which even the parents themselves are subjected.

Achievement, of course, is one of the most exhaustively researched areas of psychology. But in the long run, achievement per se is not the central point of the problem. The child's desperate reaction is not evoked simply because the parents demand achievement from him. Rather, the child reacts against the fact that the parents want only one kind of accomplishment. In their desire to do things right and to follow the maxims of their generation by producing the best children, parents often fail to encourage a variety of accomplishments within their child. They neglect his ability to make friends, to develop trust, to exercise his fantasy, et cetera. In this respect, the parents are not merely evildoers; like their child, they are victims of their own ideas.

Given the extent of child abuse, this aspect of the problem must be of concern to all people who want to study the situation and try to do something about it.

Child abuse, of course, has its own background within the family. The people who abuse children are usually parents who feel overwhelmed by the task of raising their children. If we follow the chain of events that lead to child abuse, including child murder, we discover that the following situation is quite typical: The child does something that the parents regard as wrong. The child might cry while the father is watching the Sunday sports spectacular on television. Or the child might mess up his room although the mother is proud that her house looks like one on the cover of the magazine. Or the child dirties his pants and the mother equates this accident with disobedience and uncleanliness. Or the child has been outside playing with friends and comes home late.

In all these situations, the child comes up against the parents' value systems. The particular infraction may seem petty to outside observers, but for the parents it is such a great threat that they feel compelled to react with physical force. The parents try to protect their values (respect, obedience, order, politeness, achievement, cleanliness, et cetera) from assumed infringement on the part of the child. They want to instill these values in him, but in their overreactions they go beyond their goal. The result is child abuse and death. The tragedy of all this is that the parents, who really had the best intentions, were carried away by the rigidity of their ideas. They ended up committing crimes for which public opinion brands them as monsters and strips them of their right to human dignity. The crux of the matter would be to prevent parents from feeling their values are so threatened in the first place. They need to deal with their anxieties in other ways than through force. Beating a child is not an expression of parental strength; it is a demonstration of the helplessness that the parents are not able to admit.

These are, of course, drastic examples of family warfare. But the family contains countless other points of conflict that are expressed only partially as typical family disorders. In the majority of the cases, the family background is overlooked and only the symptoms are studied. These symptoms run the gamut from fear of contact and excessive desire to achieve, to psychosomatic illness and psychoses, and, finally, to criminality. These disorders thus have a social dimension. What happens in the family is not just a family matter, but goes far beyond it. Penal institutions, for instance, should function as corrective agencies and provide the adjustment programs that the family was evidently unable to supply. This form of reeducation, of course, tends to take the form of punishment rather than positive alternatives. It thereby operates more as a kind of social revenge than as resocialization.

But it would be one-sided to look at the family only from the perspective of its shortcomings and difficulties. An approach like that would mean that treatment would be directed only at the disorders that grow out of families. It would be a hopeless battle, much like fighting a hydra that sprouts two new heads every time one head is cut off. The manifold forms of the disorders cannot be the basis for an effective process.

In Positive Family Therapy, the foreground is occupied by the vital family relationships, the game rules within the family, and the contents of family behavior as they are transmitted to the family members. All of this takes place in two ways: The family can support its members in developing both their feelings and their ability to make differentiations. The family can thus prevent severe conflicts and disorders. In addition, the family has the capacity for reintegration and self-help. These reserves must be mobilized. In the following sections of this book, we will show how it can be done. But first we want to present some examples from various cultures. These examples will demonstrate the role of the family in the development of the individual, the unfolding of his capabilities, and the possibilities for establishing interpersonal relationships.

2. The Family as Heaven

If love and agreement are manifest in a single family, that family will advance, become illumined and spiritual; but if enmity and hatred exist within it, destruction and dispersion are inevitable.

—Abdu'l Bahá

The Grand Mogul Akbar, who lived about 700 years ago, wanted to know which was mankind's innate language. To find this out, he decreed that a number of infants be separated from their parents and be raised in such a way that their caretakers would provide the necessary food and care but not speak with them or give them special attention. The results were shocking. When the children were released, they did not have a command of any language an were unable to adapt themselves to one. They were so incapable of being educated or trained that even the attempt to utilize them in the army proved to be futile (Stokvis, 1965). In a similar experiment carried out by Friedrich von Hohenstaufen, children who were raised without language and evidence of love turned out to be very vulnerable and died in a relatively short time (Mitscherlin, 1967).

Recent investigations have yielded similar results: Three groups of children, all from the same social level, were compared with each other. The first group was made up of children from normal family situations. The children in the second group were ones whose mothers were prison inmates; contact between these children and their mothers had been limited to about two hours a day. The third group consisted of children from orphanages where the care they received had met only the most basic needs. The children in this last group had the highest mortality rates, were more socially inept, and scored the lowest on intelligence tests. The children who grew up in normal families, on the other hand, did better on intelligence tests and in measurements of their physical condition. They were also proved to be less susceptible to emotional disorders (cf. Spitz, 1960, 1967; Bowlby, 1952).

Other studies (Fischer, 1952; Schenk-Danzinger, 1961; Meierhofer and Keller, 1966) demonstrated that linguistic development is hampered if maternal care is withdrawn during the first months of infancy.

From these experiments it is clear that upbringing determines the development of the individual. The family represents the basic model for the individual's socialization right from the moment of birth. He needs the family for the satisfaction of his basic needs and for the development of his capabilities. Within this basic structure there are many variations of familylike structures and institutions.

The educational contents transmitted within the family are by no means unchangeable and universally valid. As can be seen in observations by Margaret Mead (1970) and Erik H. Erikson (1971), the norms are dependent on social and cultural conditions: "Which factors in upbringing help to produce a child who is gentle, contented, good-hearted and trusting, neither aggressive, overly ambitous nor reckless?" Mead answers this question on the basis of her anthropological studies. "There is a fine and clear connection," she writes, "between the way a child is fed, put to bed, disciplined, taught to control himself, cuddled, punished and encouraged and the final product as an adult." Erikson confirms the basic findings of this study with investigations he carried out among the Bioux and Urok Indians. He paid particular attention to feeding rituals and toilet training and correlated them with the aggressive/resigned character of the Sioux and the compulsive/orderly and clean behavior of the more peace-loving Uroks. Erikson extended this comparison to encompass Western cultures in general. He writes:

> *As we will see, there are cultures where the parents ignore anal behavior and leave it up to the older siblings to lead the toddler into the bushes so that its desire to take care of the matter eventually corresponds to its desire to imitate its elders. Our Western civilization, however, has chosen to take the matter more seriously; how seriously depends on the pervasiveness of middle class morals and of the ego-ideal of a mechanized body. In such cases it is simply taken for granted that early, rigorous toilet training does more than make the atmosphere in the home more "decent." It is also absolutely essential for the development of order and punctuality. . . . Without a doubt, there is among the neurotics of our day that compulsive type whose need for mechanical punctuality and thrift in his preferences as well as with his feces is greater than is good for him and, in the long run, for society as well. In many parts of our culture toilet training has obviously become the most difficult aspect of child rearing.*

As the basic unit for socialization, the family stands right in the middle between cultural tradition and social change. The family is what produces the individual and gives him his particular stamp. It provides him with the tools he needs to exist in the group that surrounds his family. It is the juncture for interpersonal relationships and thus defines how the physical, emotional, and cognitive abilities of the individual can be developed. A person needs more than mere information for his upbringing. He also needs an emotional base so that he can become the master of this upbringing. The child needs more than stimuli for the development of his capacity for order, achievement, thrift, punctuality, and dependability. He also needs emotional warmth, security, patient attention from his parents, and ties to the other people in his surroundings. To be sure, pure upbringing can work to build character; but the person in charge can easily lose control so that it then becomes the source of conflicts., disagreements, and disorders.

Conscious upbringing is more than a matter of knowing the various contents of that education. The goal must be kept in mind at all times. One must constantly ask, "Why am I raising my child? For my own sake? For the sake of the child? For humanity?" This leads to another question: If parents teach the children, who teaches the parents? The answers to these questions decide the fate of a family and the people who live within it.

3. The Family as Fate

Even though everyone is fated to die, don't put your head in the mouth of the lion.

—Saadi (Persian poet)

The original religious concept of fate is closely related to two questions whose answers can lead to hope, despair, or fatalistic resignation. Those two questions are: "What things are unchangeable; what must one learn to bear?" and "What can a person influence, correct, or treat?"

These questions point to *fixed fate* and *conditional fate*. *Fixed fate* refers to those things that are unavoidable: Everyone is born and dies. Nothing can circumvent these events. Conditional fate, however, has its own history; it could have been avoided and was or still is subject to change. The following example can illustrate the relationship between fixed and conditional fate: A candle has a fixed fate in that its wax burns and is consumed; its eventual dying out is therefore a destiny that cannot be changed. The conditional fate, however, is comparable to the following event: While the candle is still quite tall, a gust of wind comes and extinguishes the flame. This is a question of conditional fate, since there would have been a number of ways to keep the candle from going out.

Many behavioral patterns and human characteristics frequently considered innate and fateful are really the result of events that left their mark early in childhood. This can be illustrated with an example from the animal world; namely, the fact that the tiger hunts and kills its prey. Behavioral research has shown that hunting is innate in the tiger but killing the victim is first learned from the mother. From this we can see that a mode of behavior that appear to be a single entity is made up of various components derived from many sources. In human beings, where there is even less instinctive behavior, the relationship between "innate" and "acquired" behavior must be even more complex.

If a father demands peace and quiet and nervously withdraws into himself when he comes home in the evening, not just he alone, but also his wife and children regard this as unavoidable fate. The members of the family grumblingly comply, even though they are still angry about it. No one, least of all the father, hits upon the idea that there are other ways to deal with being tired. The father, after all, had seen his own father seek isolation when he was tired. If that was the custom for him, why should it be any different now? Other alternatives, such as playing with the kids, chatting with his wife, or enjoying the company of other people, seem so alien to the man that he at first finds them utter nonsense. He would rather put up with his family's dissatisfaction than try to change his old habits. Anyway, why should he change? In spite of all the grumbling from his family, this evening ritual is an established part of the family routine. No one really questions it any more.

This is only one of many examples of family life where certain features seem to be innate, instinctive, certain, and unchanging. The same thinking can be applied to a child's messiness, a husband's infidelity, a wife's jealous faithfulness, a father's pedantry, a child's propensity for telling lies, et cetera.

Every person is born with an abundance of capabilities. Which ones develop and which ones do not depends ultimately on the conducive or inhibiting influences within the environment. The teacher and therapist cannot fall back on the assertion that a particular trait is inherited. What matters is that he recognize and make use of the opportunities that exist despite or because of the disorder.

The second area that seems to be determined by fate is the social and ecological matrix into which the person is placed. This matrix gives him certain pathways where he can move with the least possible conflict. Its laws and rules form a counterpart to his own unique and individual capabilities. Whether his capabilities come to fruition or not is not simply a question of their mere existence; it depends on whether or not the environment permits their development. In his primary human surroundings, the family, daily association with other people teaches the person a program of rules and concepts that should enable him to exist in his environment. This set of rules fuses with his personality and identity, thereby forming a second nature. We call it his second nature because it appears to be the essence of his ego, but actually it is made up of behavioral aspects adopted by him from outside sources. At first glance, his behavior might appear to be truly his alone, but a closer look reveals that he has adopted his father's authority, his mother's love for order, his siblings' sense of justice when they play, his grandfather's ties to tradition, his grandmother's industriousness and care, et cetera. Later, other formative forces begin to play a role and are likewise integrated into the ego: the influence of playmates and school, job factors, his choice of a spouse, his circle of friends, and his philosophical and religious orientation. These psychosocial ties run like threads through his entire personality, giving him unique ways for solving his problems. The various roles he fills during his life and the behavioral patterns that these roles cause him to adopt are especially important. As a friend of my children, I can relate to them differently than if I am guided by traditional paternal roles and their authoritarian obligations. Role conflicts of this nature are also considered to be determined by fate.

Daily influences in the family work much like water drops that fill a barrel until one additional drop causes it to overflow. A conversation between a mother and her two-year-old will contain a number of definite clues as to what the child may and may not do. The whole range of family relationships is played out between characteristics and expectations that eventually shape the person's attitudes toward himself and his environment. As a twenty-eight–year–old patient of mine put it, "It is my fate that people pay attention to me and like me only when I accomplish something and am considerate of them."

The possible solutions a person has at his disposal are in many ways like the point where railroad tracks split off into different directions. At a certain point, someone has to decide which direction the trail will take. The travel plan determines when this will happen. Applying this idea to the family situation means that we have to determine the travel plan for the family and the individual members. This plan will guide the person's development through a variety of influences and decisions. Knowing the plan and the conditions it sets for the family makes changes possible later on. These changes are the goal of Positive Family Therapy. This means that when we treat a particular disorder, we do more than examine the background experiences of the person and ask him about his family. We delve into the family history, with all its social entanglements. Positive Family Therapy keeps its eye on what is variable and therefore changeable. What appears to be fateful is in actuality dependent on the filters set up by the individual, family, and society, letting only certain ideas, concepts, and experiences be adopted. It is entirely a question of making the changeable thinkable. Positive Family Therapy tries to do this by looking at existing problems from the viewpoints of various relational systems. The possibilities that had seemed out of the question now seem imaginable.

All of this makes it clear that Positive Family Therapy begins with the therapist. He has to devise alternatives to situations that may even seem fateful to him; then he has to transmit these alternatives to the patient's family. This requires that the therapist not look at the family dogmatically. He must remain aware of the many forms and possibilities within the family structure.

4. Forms of the Family

The injury of one shall be considered the injury of all, the comfort of each the comfort of all, the honor of one the honor of all.

—Abdu'l 'Bahá

The family is the group that the person grows up in. It determines his relationship to himself and to other people. It forms his self-image and sets forth the possibilities and limitations of his interpersonal relationships. As the institution of his primary socialization and as the area of important emotional ties, the family occupies a special place within the subsystems of a society. But despite this special role, it must not forget the sociocultural relationships and structures that surround it. Rarely can a Robinson Crusoe survive without interpersonal relationships; a Robinson family living in a social vacuum is equally uncommon. This observation holds true everywhere. It must be kept in mind whenever attempts are made to define the family or to deal with it in a therapeutic sense.

The family can be defined in terms of the biological group comprising father, mother, and children. But we also include all the institutions that provide a substitute or alternative to the family.

According to Reyam, the term "family" is derived from the Latin word *fames* (hunger). Basically, the family is a community that offers protection and basic necessities. As a biological and social structure that wards off hunger and deprivation, it has developed its own particular forms among human beings (cf. Luban-Plozza, 1978). Although the family seems to be a timeless biological and psychosocial unit, its forms have changed over the course of human history (Levi-Strauss, 1956, 1957). But one aspect of the family has remained the same: it represents the primary environment for the development of the individual.

The *nuclear family* (cf. Thomas, 1972), made up of parents and children, is a connection uniting only two generations. It is the predominant family structure in Western society today. When grandparents and other relatives and significant people are added to this group, we call it an *extended nuclear family*.

The *complete family* corresponds to the nuclear family. It is complete when it contains father, mother, and children. If one of the parents is missing, it is known as an *incomplete family*. In 1958, every twelfth child in West Germany was growing up without a father. Approximately 20 percent of all children and adolescents lived in that kind of incomplete family. Causes included illegitimate birth, separation or divorce, death of a parent, et cetera. There is a further category called functionally incomplete families. In this group, there are two parents but career factors leave them with little time for the family. Interaction with the children is usually possible only on the weekend, and even then it is limited to a few hours.

The *grand family* is a group of blood relatives from several generations, living in one place and led by a patriarchal or matriarchal figure. Found in agrarian societies, this kind of family exercises joint ownership of land, cattle, and the means of production.

The *clan* is united by blood relationships, but does not necessarily have a single leader. Nor do its members have to all live in the same place.

In agrarian societies of earlier times, we find the *household family*. Here the family lived together as a group spanning several generations. In addition, people not related by blood (servants, journeymen, maids, et cetera) were adopted into the family community, making it both a social and economic unit.

Modern industrialization dissolved this unit into small categories, the *small family* or *single parent family*. These groups had to be very mobile and ready to adapt to the working conditions prevailing at any particular time (Weber-Kellermann, 1977).

According to Thomae (1972), one of the most important changes in the family in the past few decades has been the shift from a predominantly patriarchal family order to a structure where both parents have equal input into decision making (Wurzbach, 1954; Mayntz, 1955; Goode, 1963). In terms of total populations, these changes take place slowly and as an ever-evolving modification of existing tradition.

In the archaic structures of the family, interpersonal relationships could be carried out in a direct manner. Today, however, members of the family are likely to be separated by great distances and have less of a feeling of belonging to each other. As a result, interactions among the relatives tend to take place in fantasy and in the preconscious.

This short survey of family systems shows that they have been modified by economic and social conditions as well as by relational ties. In addition to the system of names used to define the relationships, there is a system of behavioral patterns that gives substance and security to the cohesiveness of the family. As Levi-Strauss has written: "These are stylized, obligatory behaviors, sanctioned and institutionalized through taboos and priveleges. A relational system does not consist primarily of objective ties of descent or blood relationships. It stems from the subjective ideas in man's consciousness" (Levi-Strauss, 1967, p. 66). The family's numerous functions in work and economics, law and culture, and its tasks in child rearing and socialization are not basically biological conditions, but change with the development of the entire society (Weber-Kellermann, 1977).

In this sense, we want to look at the family as a system that can be approached from many directions. We want to view it as an intermediary between social norms and the development of the individual. It gets its impulses from its social setting as well as from the individual members from which it is formed. We can understand the development of the family only if we also look at the development of society and culture. Changed conditions in society have ramifications for the family and produce new tasks that it must tackle.

5. The Family Equilibrium

The family, being a human unit, must be educated according to the rules of sanctity. All the virtues must be taught the family. The integrity of the family bond must be constantly considered and the rights of the individual members must not be transgressed. The rights of the son, the father, the mother, none of them must be transgressed, none of them must be arbitrary. Just as the son has certain obligations to his father, the father likewise has certain obligations to his father, the father likewise has certain obligations to his son. The mother, the sister and other members of the household have their certain prerogatives. All these rights and prerogatives must be considered, yet the unity of the family must be sustained.

—Abdu'l 'Bahá

The family is a totality, but it is not everything. The behavior of the individual family member depends on both the family and on other social forces. Conflicts can thus develop because of changes *in* the family as well as from outside.

Unlike the transistors and relays in an electronic calculator, the relationships among family members are not static. They are subject to changes in society and thus evolve with the individual and the group. This means that the family must constantly face new developments.

Take, for example, a fifteen-year-old girl who has had close ties with her mother and lived in harmony with the rest of her family. At some point, she develops her independence and feels the need to associate with other groups of people. Suddenly she perceives her quiet family life as oppressive. Her parents and the family unit feel threatened. This is a social process with epigenous characteristics. It marks a necessary development within the family.

The family is an open social system where outside forces can exert a positive or negative influence and where the family can likewise work positively or negatively on other systems. A mother, for example, can become terribly upset when her three-year-old proudly comes home from the playground and demonstrates that he has added the word *shit* to her vocabulary. In this instance, the mother's idea of good manners and of what a child can say and do is not determined by developments within the family but by the fact that the family associates with other groups, in this case the playmates who have chosen to dispense with the customary rules when they are alone on the playground.

Another form of possible conflict within the family again comes from outside the family and is put into operation even before the family is formed. The child naturally believes his parents have been together forever, but in actuality they found each other only relatively recently. Each of the parents has a unique set of experiences, a unique educational history, and a unique life-style. Depending on which values are deemed the most important and are firmly anchored in the affective realm, the parents are generally more or less in agreement about the values that reflect the individual's ties to family traditions. But this gives rise to the question of how successfully a marriage can integrate different systems into a unique and unchanging family style. Or do the partners cling to their own parents' programming so rigidly that they are unable to achieve a new integration? Even though they form a social unit, there may continue to be differences about what is important and unimportant. These tensions can lead to conflicts with the marriage. They can be projected onto the issue of child rearing and cause the partners to take sides in questions pertaining to values and relationships. Here is a quotation from a thirty-two–year–old housewiffe, mother of one child, who needed treatment for marital problems, sexual disorders, and skin rashes due to nerves.

> *When I'm taking a bath, I'm in my element. Cleanliness is one of the most important things for me. I learned that from my parents and I've never veered from it. For my husband it is not at all important. Sometimes I get the feeling that he grew up in a pigpen. Before he goes to bed he washes his hands and face, and that's it. At least I've gotten my son to the point where he takes a shower every day.*

The family is thus susceptible to disturbances emanating from its own developmental dynamics, from the value systems it has inherited, and from confrontations with other groups. The problem is one of determining which possibilities exist in the family and in the competence of the individual to come to terms with these conflicts. Is it possible to display some flexibility? Or does the family require that its members adhere to proscribed norms? This becomes a central issue in Positive Family Therapy.

Within the family, a number of reciprocal processes run their course. Sometimes they are expressed as behavioral disorders—that is, a communication problems or as symptoms of an illness within the inidividual.

If we examine how family events can influence the origin of disease and the course of its treatment, we are faced with the question "Who is actually sick, and who should be treated?"

6. Family Therapy: Who Should Be Treated

The quality of mercy is not strained;
It droppeth, as the gentle rain from heaven
Upon the place beneath; it is twice blessed;
It blesseth him that gives, and him that takes.

—Shakespeare

When illnesses and disorders develop within our personal communities, our consciousness usually makes use of a little trick. In our minds, we tend to set up two groups: those who caused the problem and those who are suffering because of it. Of course, we usually include ourselves in that second group. The others are the villains; they are the troublemakers, the sick ones, the ones who are making up stories. This dichotomy has a lot going for it. It makes the tangled net of problems seem clear and distinct; one's own position is protected. Medical science used this trick, too. It groups people into patients and people who accompany the patients to the doctor's office. But the limitations of this view are illustrated in the following episode:

A fifty-year-old businessman, who always gave the impression of being very proper, was having a lot of trouble with his twenty-six–year–old son. He summed up the situation by saying, "I've aged ten years." The source of the problem seemed to be the son's girl friend. The businessman thought she was capable of everything—and not just of things that were proper. He was tormented by the idea that the woman's sexual charms would enable her to wrap his "immature and inexperienced" son around her little finger. After making him dependent on her, she would take him for all he owned, and he, the father, would bear the brunt of it. The father was positive that he was right about all this. But the son continued to do as he wanted. Finally the father sent him this letter:

Dear Peter,

I've taken it upon myself to put a few thoughts down on paper. You have always been very dear to us and, despite our frequent differences of opinion, you will always remain so. It was not at all my intention to change your mind about your relationship to Miss Sch. or to force you into our kind of life-style. On the contrary, it has been a very thankless task for me to persuade you to give up an erroneous path, which can be perceived only by someone who has some distance from it. In all aspects of this situation you have been the giving person, and that's why it hits you so hard. I feel bad about that. But even if the two of you were to conduct yourselves properly, a serious relationship would be a tremendous burden for you until you have completed your professional training. Such a relationship would certainly be doomed right from the beginning. Everything that happens to you, as unpleasant as it might be from time to time, should be to your personal gain. But if you continued with your friend, you would lose all faith in yourself and in your future. Living closely with other people, particularly within a family, cannot succeed without diplomacy and compromise. Otherwise there is constant fighting and tension, and nothing can survive that. You will have to decide whether you will forever resent our intruding into your affairs, or whether you will realize that our actions stem only from our concern for you, our son. What we did, we did with the best intentions, with no thought for ourselves. You are not an object or instrument with which we can demonstrate our power. More than anything else, I want my son to be a free man with his own initiatives and freedom in how he lives his life. That's why I now say to you, "It's your life. Make the best of it." Shake off your facade and your false behavior and be the person you really are, a decent and valuable man. My son is too good to be a mere plaything in the hands of a woman with questionable intentions; too good for playful hours with someone with a suspicious background. Find your own way and you will once again be a happy person; at the same time you will also find the way to success and contentment. In the future act only according to your best interests. We don't want to and can't intervene in your affairs again. You and I are really more similar than we are willing to admit.

With Love,
Your father

The father's showing of concern for his son was not limited just to this letter. With the backing of his wife and both grandparents, he influenced his son and the girlfriend until she finally gave up. This put an end to the stumbling block, but it did not bring peace to household. Peter became apathetic. Nothing interested him anymore, not even his studies. He hung around the house like a dog on a leash. The father, feeling guilty about the whole thing, finally brought his son in for psychotherapeutic treatment.

This case history is quite typical. Through his "unreasonableness" and his depressive withdrawal, Peter had demonstrated for himself and his family who it was that was suffering, who the real patient was: he himself. This, at least, was the opinion of the family members. They agreed with the father that psychotherapy was needed, and they felt that the therapist should become their ally—and put the confused young man back on the right track and reestablish peace within the house. Without a doubt, Peter did have problems. He showed symptoms that had to be taken very seriously. But he was not the only one affected by the conflict. There was, for instance, the father. Within a short time, he took advantage of the relaxed atmosphere in the initial interview and began to describe his own problems.

He talked about how his son's affair with the woman had completely upset him. He had trouble sleeping and was plagued by terrible headaches. After all, what could have all happened if the woman had gotten control of Peter? All the influence he had acquired during his lifetime would have been on the line. How could a young man be so stubborn and keep clinging to his irrational ideas? The father himself had always listened to his parents. Their advice had served him well and had helped him become a successful man.

From these comments, the father appears to be the patient who needs help. His dilemma can be stated this way: "How can I come to terms with my son's attempts to break away from me?" Underlying this question is the father's particular ideas about thrift, achievement, and obedience—concepts that, in his opinion, represent security and the confirmation of his sense of self. Similar connections were found to exist within the other members of the family, for they, too, sought to justify themselves under the guise of being concerned about Peter. He had challenged their own values and disturbed the harmony within the family. His "misconduct" frightened them, because long-held power relationships in the family were now being threatened.

But while the symptoms and complaints give us insight into the problem, even more information is obtained through our questions about the relationships in the family, their social contacts, and their orientation to societal values: questions like "How does the son fit into the family system?"; "How do the parents treat him?"; "How do the parents get along with each other?"; "What kind of ties exist with the grandparents?"; "How do they all affect the current conflict?"; and "What are the guiding principles within the family?"

A symptom can only be understood if one knows the framework and the web of relationships in which that symptom is expressed. This is especially true for psychic and psychosomatic illnesses. Only from this point of view can one understand the role that the symptom plays within the family, within its rules of conduct, and within the social context. Like an optical illusion, the son, father, mother, and grandparents can take on the role of patient, depending on our perspective, our allegiances to the individual family members, and our opinion about who seems to be right. We are thus led to examine our ideology and the defense mechanisms we develop in response to the conflict and the parties involved.

The members of an ecological system such as that represented by the family are all elements of an interactive circle where the conduct of one individual invariably influences the conduct of all the others (Stierlin, 1977).

In all cases where mental or psychosomatic problems are noticeable, we can find these kinds of connections if we look at more than just the medical history of the person showing symptoms. We face the question of who is sick and who should be treated—the person who comes to us as the patient? Or his family, partners, superiors, colleagues, society and its institutions, the politicians who represent him and his social needs? Or should we treat the people who pose as therapists for him? All of this challenges the traditional way of dealing with the mentally ill and calls into question our institutions for psychiatric treatment.

It is no longer just a matter of applying a certain form of treatment to a certain illness, like, for example, admitting someone to a psychiatric clinic. Instead, we emphasize the inquiry into how these measures affect the patient, his family, and the course of his illness.

7. Family or Clinic

You see both have their places. Those diseases that are due to psychological neurosis, treat them according to psychological neurosis and suggestive therapeutics, and those that are due to material causes, then you have to give them the material treatment.

—Abdu'l 'Bahá

According to a report on psychiatry in West Germany (1975), about one-third of the West German people have had a mental illness at some time in their life or are still suffering from one. This amounts to approximately 20 million people. Of the 42 million Germans who see a doctor every year, between 4 and 8 million go because of mentally related problems. A million urgently need psychiatric or psychotherapeutic treatment. Every year 600,000 people go to a nerve doctor and 200,000 are admitted to a nerve clinic. These statistics say nothing about the number of patients or potential patients who seek help but find themselves trapped in the medical-psychological-psychiatric-psychotherapeutic labyrinth and do not get treatment from a specialist.

The social communities surrounding the individual are the place where conflicts develop. For the child, this community is the family he was born into. Later, it is generally the family he founds himself. But other communities, also exert an influence. As the environments in which the individual develops they pose the danger that the individual will not develop properly. How do we deal with people who seem mentally disturbed? What are the consequences of our methods of treatment? These questions are particularly crucial in the psychiatric treatment of the mentally ill.

Psychiatric practice in the late nineteenth and early twentieth centuries developed a treatment model that continues today despite much criticism. The patient is removed from his everyday environment and is put into a psychiatric clinic so that he will "recover." This raises the question as to whether this isolation is really good for the patient or if it is mainly for the benefit of the family members and other people concerned. Is isolation perhaps based on the belief that the problem is solved if the patient is put into the hands of a proficient doctor? Without a doubt, a clinic is a source of relief for a family that is suddenly faced with a mentally ill relative. Since a clinic relieves the family of the need to take care of the patient themselves, they can continue their regular work. The clinic thus represents a division of labor whereby the work force does not have to be diminished.

The usual practice of admitting the patient to a clinic for a set period of time stems from the desire to remove the patient from an environment that has become burdensome to him. But perhaps the reverse is also true. Willi (1978) makes a comparison with a greenhouse. Sickly plants are brought in and are protected from severe weather in the hope that later on they can be transplanted to the outdoors again. The transplantation of the patient is a difficult intrusion into his psychosocial system. Because of the clinic's atmosphere of warmth, support, and understanding, the patient can easily come to project all his troubles onto the outside world. Because it is so pleasant within the psychotherapeutic community, the old relationships with family and friends seem all the colder. But when the patient is taken out of his familiar surroundings, the rest of the family experiences more problems than is generally assumed. The harmony within the family is disturbed, and the conflict-laden rules continue to operate. The sick family keeps producing new patients. Another effect is that the family shields itself from the patient and emotionally rejects him as "the sick one." When it becomes absolutely necessary to admit a family member into a clinic, it is good for the family to seek help in dealing with the conflicts brought about by the patient's absence. Like other therapists, I have found that family members are more likely to be amenable to therapy if they are treated sympathetically and are presented with interpretations that are acceptable to them and at the same time give them insight into the family conflicts. Above all, they don't want the therapist to make them the scapegoat for the patient's condition.

In a concrete sense we can draw the following conclusions: The family and the social milieu should receive more attention in the therapeutic process. Psychiatric hospitals that in part function only as a kindergarten or nursery school should be transformed into outpatient clinics, therapy centers, and advisory offices where family members can be prepared for their therapeutic roles and the patients themselves can come to understand how they must participate in the therapeutic process. The patient's friends have a particular responsibility; for good or bad, they exert a direct and powerful influence. In many cases, the influence of the parents, friends, and neighbors can determine the course of the illness. The conflict can thus be visualized as a network in which the relationships between family members function as important points of contact. How can the problem be approached? The answer lies in regarding the whole family as a patient. Regardless of who occupies the limelight in the treatment, Positive Family Therapy looks at the entire family structure and includes it in the analysis.

In the last few years, family therapy has grown in importance—to become so important, in fact, that individual therapy now finds it worthwhile to examine family relationships as a part of its treatment of the individual.

8. The Development of Family Therapy

WHOM SHOULD YOU BELIEVE?

"Can you lend me your donkey for this afternoon?" a farmer asked the mullah.

"Dear friend," replied the mullah, "you know that I am always ready to give you help when you need it. My heart longs to lend my donkey to you, an orthodox man. It pleases my eye to see you bring home the fruits of the field with my donkey. But what can I say, my dear friend? At the moment, someone else has my donkey."

Moved by the mullah's sincerity, the farmer thanked him profusely by saying, "Well, even if you couldn't help me, your kind words have helped me a great deal. May God be with you, O noble, kind, and wise mullah." But, as the farmer was still frozen in a deep bow, there came from the stall a bloodcurdling heehaw. The farmer was startled, looked up in astonishment, and finally asked mistrustingly, "What do I hear? Your donkey is there after all. I heard his donkeylike voice."

The mullah turned red with anger and screamed, "You ungrateful man. I told you the donkey is not there. Whom do you believe more: the mullah or the stupid cries of an even more stupid donkey?"

Conceptually, family therapy stands in contrast to individual therapy. While the latter deals with the individual and establishes a two-party relationship between therapist and patient, the family is the essential entity for treatment in family therpay. The term "family therapy" signifies primarily a special way of setting up the therapeutic situation. It says nothing about an obligatory theory or method for family treatment. Instead of theories and methods, there are several therapeutic aspects that have developed from various points of departure. In the following pages, we will present a brief, albeit incomplete, synopsis of these developments and also describe the current state of the methods used in family therapy. In presenting this information, we will not limit ourselves to developing academic theories.

HEALING PROCESSES IN THE FAMILY

The history of family therapy began long before psychotherapy was scientifically institutionalized, in response to the social changes brought about by industrialization, the division of labor, and the disintegration of the family. Hypothetically we can say that there have been interpersonal problems and inner conflicts since the dawn of mankind. Attempts to deal with these problems have probably existed just as long. A significant portion of these occurrences took place with the family, even though its structure may have changed over the course of time.

Back then—as is generally the case today—family therapy was basically self-help. People "treated" each other by drawing on their own experiences, traditional strategies for resolving conflict, and the prevailing morality of their time. Experienced members of the family took on the role of advisors and in this capacity received acknowledgment and trust from the clan. This development expanded to include such areas as educational, marital, and family counseling. In the next stage of this process, the consultations drew on the findings of pedagogy and psychology and began to take place in public and private establishments outside the family.

RELIGIOUS-PHILOSOPHICAL INFLUENCES

The social order and its philosophical systems provided the ideological framework for self-help in the family and offered tools for handling individual and family problems. In almost all religious and philosophical systems, the family is looked upon as the norm. Marriage is considered its base. In Roman Catholic doctrine, for instance, sex is restricted to marriage and the couple's reproductive function is strongly emphasized (Bonaventure, Duns Scotus). For Augustine, marriage is given meaning by its production of offspring, its fidelity, and the indissolubility of the union (Lau, 1965). The child-parent relationship was likewise based on these rules. According to Augustine, the offspring were to be received with love, cared for with heartfelt goodness, and raised in the fear of the Lord. The Old Testament even threatens children with the death sentence if they fail to honor and obey their parents. Given this background, treatment was not to be given to the family per se but to the family members who deviated from it. Since the marriage, as a union created by God, was to remain intact regardless of the circumstances, the chief goal was to prevent one of the spouses from going off on his or her own, even if it meant that that spouse might be destroyed by staying in the marriage. Through discussion, counseling, regulations, and an inventory of punishments that would be meted out in this world and the next, society tried to correct the behavior and perhaps even relieve the individual's suffering.

ABOUT THE NECESSITY FOR FAMILY THERAPY

During the Age of Enlightenment, the religious world order retreated into the background as more emphasis was placed on the individual. As the "measure of all things," man thought about the persistence of his needs and considered how he could use his reason to establish the rules for his interpersonal relationships. The family took on a new meaning. It was no longer justified simply as being part of the divine order. Instead, it was now looked at as the result of blood ties, the fertile soil for raising children, and a bulwark against human isolation. During the Age of Industrialization, the family lost its function as the chief unit for production in agriculture and the crafts. The father, in particular, lost much of his authority, his sense of superiority, and the honor due him in old age. Horkheimer (1967) suspects that this change in the father's stature has produced the type of person who continually looks for an authority figure. Horkheimer writes; "In earlier times the source of moral autonomy was the loving imitation of the self-assured, competent man devoted to his duties. The child growing up today, having only an abstract idea of arbitrary power instead of a real father image, looks for a superfather." Mitscherlich (1963) grasps this change of structure in a uniquely dialectical concept of "fatherlessness and speaks of the "path to a fatherless society." As Horkheimer sees it, the role of the mother has undergone similar change. "The ideal modern mother," he writes, "plans the upbringing of her children almost scientifically. . . . Her entire attitude toward the child becomes rational: even love is administered like a component of pedagogical hygiene. . . . The mother ceases to be a moderating force between the child and the harsh reality. She herself becomes reality's mouthpiece" (pp. 277f.). Marcuse (1967) sees a social danger in the family's loss of power. As long as it assured an intact private realm, the family was a counterforce to the public power. Thus the shaken power within the family does not work just as a form of liberation; it also opens the way for an unbroken socialization of the child in the interest of the public power (Habermas, 1963). These pessimistic statements take on new importance when one notes that precisely in this period, when the dissolution of the family seems to pose a real threat, family therapy is receiving fresh impetus as a new method of treatment. Together with developmental psychology and social psychology, it is trying to build a new psychosocial base for understanding the family. This tendency is also contained in such seemingly contradictorily conceived views as those of Cooper (1971), who thematicizes the death of the family. Against this background the motto for family therapy seems to be "The family is dead. Long live the family!"

With the shift in emphasis from a clerical to a secular world, the physician became a specialist whose tasks involve problems, conflicts, behavioral disorders, and mental illnesses. This trend began with the family doctor or general practitioner whom people turned to because of his perceptiveness and his good advice. As psychiatry then developed as a separate branch of medicine, the close relationship between family health and psychological treatment was lost.

FROM PSYCHOANALYSIS TO FAMILY THERAPY

Under Freud's influence, the development of psychoanalysis at the turn of the century yielded new insights into psychodynamics and psychogenetic processes. Psychodynamics deals primarily with the three psychic components of the structure set forth by Freud: ego, id, and superego. These three components can be summarized as follows: The ego is a structure of the personality that referees between the other two components and reality. The id is comprised of all the desires and affects that seek a satisfaction of the drive. The superego contains the norms and moral demands accepted into the personality. From this theory we can derive essential family functions: the family as the place where needs are satisfied (id function), as the place where the conscience is informed of the behavioral norms and drives are suppressed in accordance with family and social rules (superego function), and as the place where compromises, conformity, and defenses are tested (ego function). In the psychogenetic model, the connection between the psychic apparatus and the family structures can be seen even more clearly. This model describes the development of the personality and its instinctual wishes at various stages, each of which is associated with a specific object relationship. These "object relationships" reflect aspects of the family environment that are important to the child. In the oral phase, extending over the first twelve months of life, the infant is totally dependent on his environment. His reality is limited to the mother-child relationship. The anal phase (age one to three) goes hand in hand with toilet training, motor development, and development of body control. During this phase, the child learns to adopt parental orders. In the Oedipal phase, the conflict centers on the three-sided relationship of father-mother-child. The latter wants to win the attention of the parent of opposite sex and is competing with the parent of the same sex. The needs stemming from this phase are dealt with in the family relationships according to the social norms and the morality of the family members. Important aspects of the family relationship were thus investigated, at least insofar as they affect the maturation process of the individual. The child was in the center: from the child's perspective, his family partners appear to be reduced to objects he can use to determine the direction of his impulses and establish the base for his identification needs, which are necessary for the development of his ego and superego.

Although the family relationships were important in the daily life of the patient, in his fantasy, and in the transference relationship with his analyst, one dealt with them only as imaginary dimensions. In deference to the dogma of psychoanalytic procedures, the real family was kept in the background, as if behind a curtain. Furthermore, the psychoanalytic setting tempered the family relationships. As if governed by a rule of abstinence, the analyst was not supposed to show emotional reactions such as consolation, sympathy, et cetera, nor was he allowed to give advice or express his opinions. Also, the patient was not allowed to tell a third party about what happened in the analysis. In addition, the patient was advised not to make any big decisions like marriage, divorce, or a career change while he was in therapy. Although these rules are undisputedly important for the analytic situation, they tend to isolate the patient from his family and prevent it from taking part in the therapeutic events. Analysis thus becomes a "functional clinic stay" for the patient. One function of the abstinence rule is the better control over the often-complicated transference relationships. But this can lead to a situation where an orthodox psychoanalyst fears that the entry of a further family member will cause him to lose therapeutic control. The family structures outlined in psychodynamics and psychogenesis, however, allowed psychoanalysis to pave the way for family therapy. This can be documented by Sigmund Freud's analyses and, above all, by Erikson's biographical writings and cultural comparisons.

Well-known aspects of family therapy (Richter, Minuchin, Stierlin) propagated in West Germany and the United States were developed on the foundations of psychoanalytic theory, with contributions from communication theory, social psychology, and sociology and are now independent therapeutic approaches.

THE FAMILY AS SYSTEM

Models derived from communication theory, systems theory, and cybernetics provided new impulses for family therapy. According to these models, the family is a self-regulating system that functions according to rules it developed in the course of time. As Watzlawick, Beavin, and Jackson (1969) have determined, every act is a form of communication. This communication necessarily evokes a response, which again fulfills a communicative function. It is thus impossible not to communicate. This state of affairs forms the background for disorders in the family. "Families where one or more members display conduct that is traditionally diagnosed as 'pathological' are regulated by transactions (relational patterns) which are tailored precisely to this kind of pathology" (Selvini et al., 1977, p. 13). According to this paradigm, the members of the family are looked at as elements of an interactional circle. The behavior of one member influences the behavior of all of them. As a system, the family makes use of two seemingly contradictory functions: a) the tendency toward homeostasis and b) the ability to change. Homeostasis means that the family system allows only limited space for change. Jackson (1957) applied the concept of family homeostasis to the clinical discovery that the improvement of symptoms in a schizophrenic patient often has drastic effects on the family. It represents a disturbance in the family's balance and creates an imbalance that can be corrected only if another member of the family begins to show the symptoms. While homeostasis is indeed a powerful force, a family also has within it the ability to change. This goes back to its adaptive abilities. A therapeutic change is brought about by a change in the rules within the family system. "When one has realized that the symptoms are part of the transactions characteristic of the family system, there is no choice but to change the rules if one wants to change the symptoms" (Selvini et al., 1977, p. 13). An endangered communication is often characterized by rules that allow "games without an end." An example of this is the double bind, which Stierlin has translated as a "relational trap" and Loch (1961) as a "jam." It is typical for a double bind (Bateson et al., 1975) that in a crucial context various pieces of incompatible information are provided that give the partner the illusion of having alternatives. An adolescent with ambivalent dependency on his overprotective mother receives from her in various forms the challenge "Be yourself." This appeal at first seems to contradict her own unacknowledged interest in maintaining the close ties with her son under all circumstances. Aside from the anxieties and guilt feelings that this appeal can unleash, it poses this dilemma: If the son acts spontaneously, he has simply followed his mother's command and was thus not really acting spontaneously. On the other hand, he doesn't act spontaneously if he tries to act contrary to what his mother has suggested. In other words, regardless of what he does, there is no way he can be spontaneous and independent (Watzlawick, Weakland, and Fisch, 1975). These games without an end have to be ended therapeutically by using countergames. One of these paradoxical countergames is the symptom prescription (Bateson). The patient is given the task of voluntarily calling forth the symptoms that he has perceived as being uncontrollable and autonomous. As in the case of the "be spontaneous paradox," the symptom is thus no longer spontaneous. The patient steps outside the framework of his symptomatic game without an end. Selvini Palazzoli et al. (1977) describe a therapy model where this paradox and counterparadox are used to treat a family with schizophrenic disorders. Similarly, the structural family therapy developed by Minuchin (1977) is based on the theory of systems. Minuchin uses organizational structures to analyze the ordering of individual subsystems within the family system. He then uses newly structured measures to challenge the family to undergo a therapeutic change. The system-theoretical aspect for understanding the family can be extended outwardly. Speck and Attneave (1973), for instance, have added friends and associates to the nuclear family for therapy within the network of relationships. The ecological point of view (Auerswald, 1973) represents another extension of family therapy. Auerswald's perspective is interdisciplinary, including in its scope not just the family, but also the social institutions (doctor, clinic, social worker) to which the family has significant ties.

BEHAVIORAL FAMILY THERAPY

For a long time, behavioral therapy appeared to be a typical representative of individual treatment. Its process, the systematic desensitization in the treatment of fears, was tailored to the needs of the individual patient. Nonetheless, from early on behavioral therapy pointed to the social learning and the reward and punishment mechanisms that exist in a group or family. At this point, we find the beginning of a family therapy with a behavioral orientation. Libermann (1973) summarizes the basic points of this process: "Instead of rewarding inappropriate behavior by paying attention to it, family members can learn to recognize and reward a desired pattern of conduct" (p. 398). The starting point for the therapy is the reinforcing contingencies as the way the family members get along with each other. Social reinforcements include verbal and nonverbal communication, attention, and recognition: "Often the deviant family member receives a lot of sympathy or social reinforcement directed toward his inappropriate behavior and thus becomes dependent on it. The deviant person gets the message 'As long as you continue with this undesired behavior, we will be interested in and worried about you.' The recognition of such messages leads to the perpetuation of the symptomatic or undesirable behavior and to characterological patterns of activity and identity" (p. 399). Along with social reinforcement, learning from the model has particular significance for a family therapy based on learning theory. In general terms, it corresponds to imitation or identification.

As the three main tasks of the therapist, Libermann lists:

(1) The creation and maintenance of a therapeutic alliance with the patient (cf. Tausch, 1974)
(2) The establishment of a behavioristic analysis of the problems. A practical model for this is, e.g., interactional analysis as set forth by Innerhofer (1978).
(3) The expansion of the behavioristic principles of reinforcement and of model learning in the context of a continuing interpersonal interaction. Deidenbach (1978) recommends an ecologically oriented model for this.

POSITIVE FAMILY THERAPY

The development of family therapy has opened up a new dimension for psycho- and milieu therapy. The real progress in this development is that man is no longer seen as an isolated being but—in accordance with his social being—within the social ties that shape his primary existence.

Family therapy is itself a pragmatic and practice-oriented approach (cf. Haley, 1973; Ferber and Ranz, 1973). This makes it possible to regard the discrepancies between theories as being of secondary importance. Instead, we give our main attention to the commonalities and the complementary possibilities in the various psycho- and family therapy methods. Going beyond the meaning it has as an independent method of family therapy, Positive Family Therapy seeks to integrate the other theoretical and practical views and to establish connections with them. This means that Positive Family Therapy can look at these other approaches as complementary or alternative possibilities in a therapy plan (cf. Peseschkian, 1977). Before describing our Positive Family Therapy, we would like to give a brief sketch of our therapeutic conceptions: For family therapy, the family is the central relational dimension in the treatment. It is important to us to mobilize the potential for self-help inherent in every person, in every family, and even in every interpersonal relationship.

We want to develop in the family and its members the competence that is usually attributed to only the small group of psychotherapists—namely, the competence to deal with problems and conflicts in a differentiated, mature way.

9. What Does Positive Family Therapy Deal With?

If you want to put the country in order, first put the province in order. If you want to put the province in order, you have to first bring order to the cities. To bring order to the cities, you must bring order to the family. If you want to bring order to the family, you must first bring order to your own family. If you want to bring order to your own family, you must bring order to yourself.

This old saying from the Middle East describes the relational connections we live in. We have to start with the proposition that small changes in one area of life can influence the entire system. As Confucius would say, every person is responsible for the rise and fall of humanity. One corrupt official, for example, can discredit an entire social institution and even shake the people's faith in their social structure. Usually this is not an isolated incident and the entire society is considered to be corrupt. The corruption then becomes more or less accepted as a semilegal way of dealing with all officials.

On the other hand, changes in the entire system influence the conditions surrounding the family and the individual. An example of this is the new divorce law in West Germany, which has brought widespread change to the situation of many families. To this extent, we do indeed follow the wisdom of the Mideast. But while the Mideast idea refers to the individual as the base for all changes, as in the saying "Whoever is good to himself is good to everyone," we believe change can come from many areas. With such units as the individual, family, and society, we are really dealing with systems that are closely related to each other. Given this all-encompassing situation, one might well ask why we make the family the center of Family Therapy. It would be equally appropriate to focus on social change or the isolated treatment of an individual. But let's recall what we have already said about the family. As the site for biological and social reproduction, it occupies a unique and central role in the events within society. If we ask about the source of a person's unique qualities, views, and values, we probably end up talking about the environment he grew up in—namely, his family. In addition, the continuity of society depends on rules that one acquires within the family and on the common values that hold the society together.

Along with these functions there is another important one. In his first few years of life, man is particularly malleable. The child has an abundance of capabilities that are still relatively unformed and undifferentiated. Even if they are not evident, they are present. These capabilities will unfold in certain ways, depending on the people around the child and the developmental opportunities that his family offers. In some instances, the capabilities will be suppressed or will develop in an imbalanced way. The emotions within a family, not only ones like trust and hope, but also mistrust, despair, and aggression, are expressed primarily toward people one is most closely tied to. These people are generally one's parents, siblings, children, spouse, and members of the extended family such as grandparents, uncles, aunts, et cetera. This strong emotional involvement, plus the fact that one spends a lot of time within the family, make it a particularly important group. Conflicts can both emerge and be solved there.

Family therapy looks at the family as a system. It is of secondary importance which element in the system is changed, just as long as the change is looked at in a therapeutic sense. In practice, this means that Positive Family Therapy must not be based on a particular psychotherapeutic dogma. It is more important that there be several ways of giving shape to the process. All of them can be described as family therapy and are described as follows.

WORK WITH THE INDIVIDUAL PATIENT

At first glance, it seems paradoxical to label this as family therapy. But from a pragmatic point of view, this process is necessary if the other parties in the conflict cannot be included in the therapeutic sessions. In accordance with the belief that one change in a system's elements can influence the entire system, the patient in Positive Family Therapy is given the task of dropping his patient role and functioning as a therapist in his own situation. Experience shows that a family's initial opposition to therapy can be broken down and the entire family can eventually be included in the process. Furthermore, the patient's role change from patient to therapist ushers in a change of behavior and thus having therapeutic effects on the whole family.

Even in typical individual therapy we must not lose our orientation toward family therapy. I have found that a considerable percentage of the individual patients had sought therapy at the advice or insistence of their families. These were delegated patients sent out by their families. In contrast to the family members who stayed at home, these patients often had the courage to demand help from therapy.

In individual therapy there develops the classic therapist-patient relationship in which the patient, by using his memory, can summon up the family relationships mirrored in his experience. The family is thus present as an imagined and reexperienced entity, ready to be interpreted and evaluated for the patient. But in Positive Family Therapy we don't just draw on an analysis of the problems of transference; we also stimulate the patient's intuitive associations through the use of particular themes and stories (cf. Peseschkian, 1979).

WORK WITH PARTNER GROUPS (COUPLE THERAPY)

These groups are a particular type of family group. The couple together seeks the services of a therapist. Problems in their relationship or in the environment—children, in-laws, work, et cetera—can become the objects of the therapy. Both partners come to the session together, and in their conduct there they provide the therapist with a sample of how they interact with each other. The therapist can intervene directly and try to change their behavior, or he can lead them to a cognitive differentiation of the conflict and help them become aware of the opportunity they have to change their patterns of interaction.

Anyone with even a bit of experience in couple therapy will know that most couples in therapy are under tremendous pressure when they talk about their conflict. Discussing the problem, they are likely to feel like tearing each other apart. In Positive Family Therapy, we don't immediately jump into the lions' den and start talking about the conflict. Instead, we begin by discussing the things that hold the couple together and what function the conflict is having in their relationship. We thus create a common ground for dealing with the conflictual contents. This puts the partners in a new situation where they can look for new ways of solving their problems. Of course, sometimes divorce or separation is the solution they finally decide upon.

WORK WITH THE NUCLEAR FAMILY

Here we look at the family in a narrow sense of the term. The father, mother, and those children who are still living with their parents are present. The experience of the conflict and its solution are carried out, as far as possible, within the original family situation. One of the advantages of this process is that one can observe the rules governing how the family members interact with each other. These patterns of interaction can then be described as concepts. The father, for instance, might try to control the communication by answering for the other members of the family. In individual therapy, we work with the patient's perceptions of his family, but in family therapy we have direct access to the family's concepts and rules and thus have more opportunity to deal with them through direct intervention. But we do not rely solely on direct intervention, as is the case with family therapy based on systems theory. Instead, Positive Family Therapy uses a five-stage intervention system to identify both the family rules and their conceptualizations. The family then receives this tool as an aid in self-help. It helps the family members clarify and differentiate their own positions and makes them more aware of misunderstandings. Individual techniques related to this process are discussed in the following chapter. At this point, it should be noted that the therapeutic process shifts from therapy per se into the area of self-help. The patients learn at an early stage of their therapy that they can free themselves from the therapy situation and use the instruments at hand to work through conflicts on their own. Therapeutic skills are thus transferred to the patient-family and its members.

WORK WITH THE EXTENDED FAMILY

In addition to the nuclear family, other closely related people can take part in the treatment: grandparents, uncles, aunts, close friends of the family, et cetera. The size of the group is limited only by organizational restrictions. Now more than ever, the living history of the concepts begins to play an important role.

While the "family tree" of the concepts—that is, the developmental history of family attitudes and rules—is usually discovered only through the experiences and memory of the patient, it takes on a real shape here. The therapist, as director, regulates the unfolding of the dynamic processes within the family. First he has to create an atmosphere in which the family can deal with the problems. As an impartial bystander (M. Stierlin, 1977), the therapist gives each family member the feeling of being a valuable person. Following Boszornenyi-Nagy's model (1975), he strives for an equalization of justice in the relationships among the family members. The goal of this process is to mobilize the family's reserves of those forces that lead to self-healing. Positive Family Therapy works with family concepts in which important relational rules and values have been struck down. These can now be taken up as subjects of discussion in the therapy session without inflicting injury on particular members of the family. I believe this careful process is the main reason why grandparents, for instance, who sometimes seem the least capable of change, have been able to work well in Positive Family Therapy and have benefited from it.

THE ECOSYSTEM

Here we go beyond the confines of the family. Outside contacts and social institutions now enter the therapy as intervening variables. Examples are kindergarten teachers, probation officers, colleagues, employers and supervisors, physicians, clinic personnel, et cetera. All the people and institutions that are important to a person can be approached directly or indirectly. The system to be used in therapy can be modified to include such other subsystems as institutions at one's workplace and social and governmental groups. This process supplements the family therapy and acknowledges the fact that the family is not an independent, isolated entity, but is itself part of an ecological connection. This point of view goes along with community psychology, which has as its goal the highest possible level of psychological health for the entire population. It places the main emphasis on primary prevention—that is, the prevention of psychological injuries in the first place. It thus tries to develop the individual's ability to deal with concrete situations in his daily life (cf., Sommer et al., 1978). Community psychology differs from the psychotherapist's customary practice of waiting until patients come to him for help. This practice really establishes the limits of this kind of psychotherapy, for it is unable to treat those people who for some reason or another have no access to a therapist. But community psychology tries to go beyond this limitation by actively going to the patients themselves. By doing this, it becomes involved in familial, educational, and marital counseling and also deals with work-related risks to physical and mental health.

In this sense, Positive Family Therapy sees itself as "Ecotherapy." At the present time, Positive Family Therapy does not have a tested model of community psychology. But it does try to adopt the principles of community psychology in the treatment of individuals, couples, and families. Furthermore, we see a number of possibilities for integrating the instruments of Positive Family Therapy into community psychology, thereby opening up new approaches that can be used in practice. And looking at things from the reverse direction, we see that every therapy represents an intrusion into an ecological system. Thus a social or political effect can be achieved through family therapy and even through the treatment of an individual patient. Positive achievements for the ecosystem can include such things as better adaptiveness among the people, the release from family and social entanglements, and increased ability to work productively and respond positively to one's surroundings. The importance of these changes can be assessed only in light of the society's ideology and value systems.

In connection with ecotherapy, it is worthwhile to inquire about all the general resources for self-help that exist, for instance, in the prescientific "folk psychotherapy" (cf. Peseschkian, 1977).

The ultimate goal is to develop sensitivity to the effects of one's own behavior and then to use this knowledge for one's own psychohygiene. This goal acknowledges the fact that problems and conflicts do not generally originate in therapy itself but in the person's everyday life, within his family and in his work.

Positive Therapy thus approaches all those who deal with the problems of health: psychotherapists, physicians, psychiatrists, social workers, nurses, and health administrators. Beyond these groups, it also speaks to teachers, lawyers, businessmen, private tutors, parents, adolescents, children, and everyone else who does not shut his eyes to the problems of interpersonal relationships.

POSITIVE FAMILY THERAPY TRIES TO TAKE ALL LEVELS INTO CONSIDERATION

Positive Therapy is not so much concerned that the therapist work through conflicts with a particular patient or that the therapist directly or indirectly leads the patient to a particular solution. The therapist is not primarily concerned with an isolated individuality of this kind. His partners are the members of a family and the family as a living organization. The family is stimulated to work through the existing conflicts, to test alternative behaviors, and thus to prepare possible solutions. In contrast to traditional family therapy, where the family or at least some members of the family have to be present, Positive Family Therapy views the family aspect as being already guaranteed by the fact that the family reality, as it runs its course in one's perceptions of it and in interpersonal relationships, is taken into consideration. In this sense Positive Family Therapy runs the gamut from individual treatment to community psychology, with its attention to social institutions. Regardless of where one begins, the family is still in the center: as the original group in which the individual experienced his socialization and as the place where he shapes his current emotionally important relationships.

We therefore do not simply proceed as if we are using a microscope to observe the various motives and drives that move the individual. Instead, we also use the macroscopic observation as our point of departure. The macroscopic process is akin to what takes place in sociology and social psychology, comparative cultural psychology, group and milieu psychology, and family psychology. In all of them, transactions and interactions are carefully observed. The microscopic process uncovers what goes on in the individual, i.e., events that are traditionally revealed in psychoanalysis or depth psychology. Although the sequence for using the various magnifications has not been established, we must keep all these possibilities in mind if we want to arrive at a real understanding of a person.

The applicability of customary processes of family and psychotherapy is limited because of existing barriers to communication. Up until now, these barriers have kept a large part of the population from making use of psychotherapy. The problem of the language barriers receives a lot of attention in Positive Family Therapy.

Part IV:

The Tools of Positive Family Therapy

A METAPHOR FOR THE POSITIVE PROCESS

The positive process can be compared to the following situation: A man discovered that he was in debt. This realization made it impossible for him to get any sleep. He became very depressed and wanted to commit suicide. He complained about it to a good friend. The friend listened patiently as the man told of all his problems, but when he replied, he made no mention of the debts. This surprised the man very much. Instead of discussing the debts, the friend talked about what the man owned, about his money, and about the friends who were ready to help him. Suddenly the disturbed man saw his problems in a new light. When he stopped wasting his energy on problems and debts and concentrated on the abilities he actually had, he discovered he had enough power and resources to solve his problem.

1. The Three Pillars of Positive Family Therapy

What a piece of work is man! How noble in reason! how infinite in faculties! in form and moving, how express and admirable in action, how like an angel! in apprehension, how like a God!

—Shakespeare

Since 1968 I have been working on a new concept of self-help and psychotherapy, which I call Positive Psychotherapy. The principles and techniques of this method are explained in detail in my book *Positive Psychotherapie: Theorie und Praxis einer Neuen Methode*. Now I would like to discuss how this concept can be applied within the framework of family therapy.

THE POSITIVE STARTING POINT

While many of the psychotherapeutic procedures in use today begin with disorders and illnesses, preventive medicine and psychotherapy call for a method that includes the person's abilities and developmental possibilities as well as his disorders. Through its involvement with elementary human capabilities, the basic capabilities and the actual capabilities, Positive Family Therapy is in a good position to treat people from various social classes and to illuminate transcultural problems. This starting point presupposes an answer to the two questions:

What do all people have in common?
In what ways are they different?

We try to describe general concepts of medicine, psychotherapy, and psychiatry in terms of Positive Family Therapy, to make new ways of thinking accessible to the patient, and to provide the stimulus for a new orientation within therapy and self-help.

In Positive Family Therapy, the patient gives up his old role as the patient and becomes aware of the possibilities available to him for self-help. The positive process allows us to accentuate the common grounds for understanding within the family and thus to produce a basis for the therapy. This then enables us to deal with the family disorders in a systematic way.

THE PROCESS WITH REGARD TO CONTENTS

It is generally the case that functional and dynamic connections are given careful attention in psychotherapeutic, psychological, and pedagogical literature. We, however, have made it our task to critically and systematically examine the contents of education (upbringing), of inner conflicts, and of conflicts between people. In other words, people generally tend to ask about *how* something happens (conflict process). *What* happens and the contents that determine it have until now been tangential subjects, treated at best as arbitrarily selected examples. Our inquiry into the content causes and conditions for disorders led to the actual capabilities and concepts. It is a matter of working out the family's game rules, which give special meaning to physical and mental symptoms and determine how the family tends to deal with conflicts that might arise. This process of looking at the game rules thus enables us to accomplish two things. We can identify the family's existing capacity for self-help and at the same time work through the conflicts in the family.

THE FIVE/STAGE POSITIVE FAMILY THERAPY

An additional motivation for our work was the need for a conflict-centered therapy that is as efficient and effective as possible. This strategy is divided into observation-distancing, inventory, situational encouragement, verbalization, and broadening of goals. The "five stages" are a model that shows how psychotherapeutic directions—even ones that differ greatly—can work together.

The following chapters describe the tools of Positive Family Therapy that can be applied in the therapeutic situation and as

means of self-help. The three pillars of Positive Family Therapy will be described separately, even though they are inseparable in therapeutic practice. While looking at the positive aspects of an illness or disorder, we give the patient and his family the opportunity to relinquish the symptom and grapple with the conflict behind them. This conflict is described in terms of its contents. The five stages of Positive Family Therapy help find a way to go from the conflict itself to ways of dealing with it.

2. The Positive Starting Point

ABOUT THE CROW AND THE PEACOCK

In the palace park, a black crow perched on the branches of an orange tree. Down on the well-tended lawn, a peacock marched around proudly. The crow screeched, "How can one even permit such a strange bird to enter this park? He walks around as arrogantly as if he were the sultan himself. And with those downright ugly feet! And his feathers such a horrible shade of blue! I would never wear a color like that. He drags his tail around like a fox." The crow stopped and waited silently for a reply. The peacock did not say anything for a while, but then he began to speak with a mealncholy smile. "I don't think your assertions correspond to reality. The bad things you say about me rest on misunderstandings. You say I'm arrogant because I hold my head up so that my shoulder feathers stick out and a double chin disfigures my neck. In reality, I'm anything but arrogant. I know my ugly features, and I know my feet are wrinkled and like leather. This actually bothers me so much that I hold my head erect in order not to see my ugly feet. You see only my ugly parts. You close your eyes to my fine points and to my beauty. Haven't you noticed that? What you call ugly is exactly what people admire in me."

—after P. Etessami, Persian poet

Patients don't simply suffer from their illnesses and disorders, but also from the hopelessness that is suggested to them by the diagnosis itself. This state of affairs is historically and culturally determined. As a result, the description of human capabilities and disorders is not based solely on one model; it can include other models of thought derived from other people's behavior, other theoretical constructs, and other cultures.

THE WITHOUT/EVIDENCE PRINCIPLE

A considerable part of human awareness takes place according to the nonic principle: How something really is remains unmentioned; in its place, one expresses what is not. When a person is asked how his job is, he tends to reply, "Not bad." This answer leaves much unsaid. In a similar way, traditional psychotherapy derives its image of man from psychopathology. It describes disorders and illnesses and implies that health will be restored if these disorders are corrected.

There is some truth to this view, for only in rare cases does a patient go to a therapist just to have his health confirmed. More likely, the patient goes to him to be cured of his illness. In accordance with this idea, medicine has developed the Without-Evidence principle, with the consequence that the illness is treated, not the patient. The illness thus emerges like a dark cloud between the therapist and the patient. It becomes the focus of the therapist's attention. The patient quickly learns that he can get the therapist's attention only by virture of the illness. Thus the illness looms more and more strongly in the foreground and the exclusive preoccupation with negatively colored experiences leads to a repetition of the illness and the patient's neurotic ideas. On the cognitive level, this means that the patient continues to act according to ideas that typify his disordered way of dealing with conflict.

An example of this is the choice of symptoms, an area where the therapist also has some input. In the total picture of a psychosomatic illness, it is rare that there is only one symptom. Most of the time, there are several different symptoms running parallel to each other, but the therapist in charge of the treatment will focus on one particular group of symptoms. A patient suffering from heart trouble and depression will be viewed in different ways: An internist will examine and treat primarily the heart condition, while a psychiatrist deals with the depression. At the same time, each specialist provides the patient with his views about the illness and his particular interpretation of the symptoms. Take, for example, the following different responses given to a female patient. Despite their disparate sources, they all repeated the somatic attitude.

The patient, thirty-two years old, was suffering from anxiety, stomach problems, headaches, inner unrest, and pains in her shoulders and arms. The treatment first began with the internist's attention to her stomach problems. In a transitional episode, an orthopedist treated her shoulder and arm pains by using ultraviolet rays. A psychiatrist then prescribed tranquilizers and antidepressants for her depression and anxiety. But then the woman's headaches drove her to a neurologist, who diagnosed a trigeminus neuralgia. The patient seemed satisfied with this diagnosis until her internist referred her to a psychotherapist two years later. In the course of the therapy, it was discovered that all her symptoms could be traced back to a mental conflict that had assumed a somatic form.

The external events accompanying her conflict included marital problems, the death of her beloved brother, and the loss of her job. The patient suppressed the conflict, but reacted by producing the previously mentioned symptoms. This physical reaction enabled her to gain the support of the physicians treating her. Only the internist, with his interest in psychotherapy, saw the connections between the symptoms and made it possible for her to begin a successful treatment that uncovered the roots of her problem.

LEARN TO MAKE DISTINCTIONS

In my therapeutic practice, I am frequently confronted with a misunderstanding. If a child has fever, a headache, stomach pains, or a heart ailment, we treat that child with special care. But if, in our eyes, the child acts "funny,"—i.e., different that what we are used to—or even impolite and unruly, our tolerance reaches its limits quite quickly. In other words, we react in a negative or aggressive way. We too often overlook the fact that the behavior could have the characteristics of an illness. There are definite consequences of our tendency to place more value on physical illnesses: If one feels ill, one is inclined to go to a doctor. But one seldom thinks about consulting a therapist, even when it is a clear case of psychic disorders.

Does one have to be divorced in order to realize for the first time how good marriage is? Does one have to suffer a heart attack to be convinced of how important physical health can be? Does one have to know someone who commited suicide to understand the importance of mental health? Does one have to have sat in jail to know how wonderful freedom is? Does one have to turn his car into a pile of junk to know that driving recklessly in heavy traffic carries a big risk?

Conflicts and disorders, as a rule, originate in everyday life, not in psychotherapeutic practice. Marital problems, for example, develop initially out of the partners' relationship and in connection with their other social contacts. In the case of infidelity on the part of a spouse or lover, for instance, there are other ways to react besides seeking "justice" and the restoration of "honor" with a gun or knife. One can drown his sorrows in alcohol; one can try to find a better world by taking drugs; one can get back at the partner by also being unfaithful. But one can also seize the opportunity and tackle the problem in an active way. All of this is self-help.

But some forms of self-help have the disadvantage of provoking even more trouble and anger. It is ultimately a matter of finding measures that are acceptable and feasible for both partners. This book points to such methods.

3. What Is "Positive Family Therapy"?

The healthy person is not one who is free of problems, but one who is in a position to deal with them.

—Tenet of Positive Psychotherapy

The term "positive" is usually used as a moral categroy. Regardless of the value judgment designated as "positive," it depends on the value system, which sets the standards for good and bad.

This relational system is what positive family therapy investigates. Here *positive* takes on an additional meaning. As in its original usage (Latin *positum*), it refers to what is factual and given. Factual and given things are not necessarily conflicts and disorders, but also the capabilities inherent in every human being. We don't mean that everything should be looked at in a positive light; rather, Positive Family Therapy tries to differentiate between the critical behavior and the capabilities. Only through this process can we separate stable, less conflictual behavioral components from the symptoms. This process prepares the patient and his environment to deal with existing problems in more effective ways.

The ability to make differentiations is basic to all our physical, mental, and social functions. Therapeutic intervention, regardless of the particular method used, is ultimately an attempt to make it possible for the patient to make more precise and appropriate distinctions. This ability enables him to respond to the demands of a situation in ways appropriate to his own particular goals.

According to traditional views, the illness stands between the therapist and the patient:

Therapist	Illness	Patient

Traditional Process

As soon as we concentrate on the regenerative powers of the patient instead of exclusively on his illness, the relationship between the therapist and the patient takes on a new quality:

Therapist	Capabilities Illnesses	Patient

Positive Process

The principles underlying education, treatment, and psychotherapy have always been dependent on the image of man generally accepted in that particular era. This image of man is comprised of the experiences one has with his own parents and fellowmen as well as the experiences common to his social tradition or adopted from other ones. These experiences can vary from group to group and, in a larger sense, are dependent on the value system set forth by the prevailing philosophy or religion.

In earlier times, particularly in classical Greece, the psychically ill person was revered, for it was thought that he had a special connection to the world of the gods. In the early Christian era, society developed a sense of pity for the mentally ill. As the outcast and stigmatized, they seemed to wear Christ's crown of thorns. In medieval Europe, however, the mentally ill were thought to be possessed by devils and demons. Attempts were made to drive out the devils through exorcism, beatings, enemas, et cetera. Often the mentally ill were locked up in insane asylums, put in chains, or banished as witches. At the end of the nineteenth century, when scientific methods became more accepted and doctors looked to physical causes for psychic disorders, people began to believe that environmental conditions were the root of the problem. In fact, considerable progress was made during this time as various ideas about illness were developed. Classic psychiatry is based on discoveries stemming from this period.

Along with these developments, interest came to be focused on the significance of personal experiences and the influence of the social environment in the home, school, and society. Out of this came a psychotherapeutic way of thinking that sought to change behavior and experience through psychic means. Pioneers like Sigmund Freud discovered the cause of neurotic disorders in the psychosocial conditions of the time. Eventually people began to study psychosomatic disorders and even psychoses from the perspective of psychosomatic assumptions.

From the multiplicity of schools and the disorders treated, there developed a series of methods: individual treatment, group treatment, analytic therapy, psychotherapy based on depth psychology, behavior therapy, et cetera.

4. The Positive Image of Man—Unity in Diversity

You are the fruits of one tree and the leaves of one branch.
—From the Baha'i faith

The concept of Positive Family Therapy is based on the view that every human, without exemption, possesses two basic capabilities: the ability for knowing (cognition) and the ability for loving. Both capabilities belong to the essential nature of every person. Depending on the circumstances surrounding his body, his environment, and the times (and the spirit of the times) he lives in, these basic capabilities will become differentiated and thus lead to an unmistakable structure of character traits.

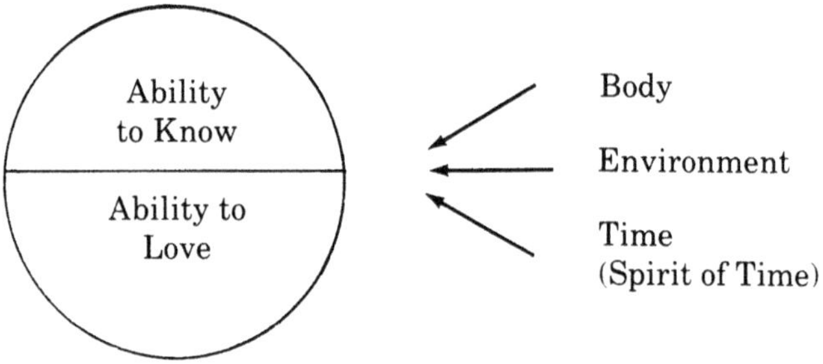

The Basic Capabilities and Their Conditions for Development

BASIC CAPABILITIES AND ACTUAL CAPABILITIES

Psychology without religion or without a philosophy of life just does not exist, in the strict sense of the word. Whenever we try to define the subject of psychology, i.e., the human being, we apply, mostly without noticing it, standards obtained from a certain philosophy of life. For instance, man is seen as a machine that reacts to certain impulses or as a creature with drives that must be continually kept in check by means of the social norms. He is seen as a product of his heritage, as having free will, or as the product of his environment. We treat a person according to how we see him. This alone makes it *necessary* for us to recognize the philosophical and religious backgrounds of our picture of man.

BASIC CAPABILITIES

The basis for the concept of Positive Psychotherapy as a metapsychology is the idea that every person, independent of his present stage of development, age, sex, race, class, typology, diseases, or social "abnormalities," possesses two basic capabilities: the capability "to know" (perception) and the capability to love (emotional sphere).

> *a) Capability to Know (Perception): Every person tries to perceive the connection within reality. He questions why an apple falls to the ground, why a tree is growing, why the sun shines, why there are sickness and sorrow. He is interested in knowing who he is, where he comes from, such questions and to look for their answers—are the capability of perception. In education, perception develops with the supply of knowledge. From there, the secondary capabilities develop: punctuality, orderliness, cleanliness, politeness, honesty, and economy.*
>
> b) *Capability of Love: The development of the capability of perception influences the success or failure of a person. The capabilities from which these experiences derive belong to the emotional sphere of the individual, the sphere of feeling, which may be called his emotional relations, an expression of his capability to love. The capability to love leads in its further development to primary capabilities like patience, time, contact, confidence, trust, hope, faith, doubt, certainty, and unity.*

These two basic capabilities develop before any cultural influence, and later the actual capabilities (the primary and secondary capabilities) develop in interaction with the three parameters of body, environment, and time.

The actual capabilities are imparted by religious, cultures, ancestors, parents, and cultural instances (school, society, and moral institutions). The capabilities of perception and of love, however, belong to the nature of every human being. This means simply that man—in his original nature—is good.

Unity in Diversity

Just as a seed contains an abundance of capabilities that are unfolded through interaction with the environment—soil, rain, the gardener—man develops his capabilities through his close relationships with the world around him. This is why we don't encounter the two basic capabilities in a pure sense but in the forms they have adopted through the relational structures in the family and society and through experiences in the person's life. All other capabilities (cf. actual capabilities) develop out of the basic capabilities and the particular unfolding within their environment.

The hypothesis of the basic capabilities means nothing more than: *Man is essentially good.* This holds true regardless of race, social class, or psychological type. The basic capabilities are not limited solely to the healthy people; they are equally present in the sick person, whose physical and mental functions are disturbed. If these capabilities are inhibited, neglected, or developed in an imbalanced way, there are susceptibilities to conflicts—either hidden or apparent.

In other words, there are no persons who are inherently bad. If we can't stand someone, it might be because we don't like his looks. If we detest someone, become upset over him, and try to keep our distance from him, it can be because his views are different than ours, or perhaps he doesn't treat us politely enough, always keeps us waiting, is unreliable, or makes demands that make us uneasy. If we don't like a person, it might be due to the fact that he disappointed us once so we don't feel we can rely on him. But we can't hate an ugly person because he is ugly, an impolite person because he is impolite, or an unreliable person because he is unreliable. Some people whom we find ugly are beautiful in the eyes of someone else. People who seem impolite to us might not have learned the kind of politeness that we expect, or perhaps their politeness is such that we have not yet come to understand. People whom we no longer trust might well deserve our confidence in other areas or at another time. Even the stage of civilization has nothing to do with man's essence. Our forefathers ate with their fingers, did not wear clothes, had no indoor plumbing, and didn't go to grade school, let alone the university. But they were nonetheless human beings, equal to us despite all the historical differences, just as people living in other cultures today represent different norms but are basically the same as we are. Even we, to cite an example, had to learn such things as cleanliness, punctuality, and efficiency—all things we are proud of. And along with them, we learned the conflict susceptibilities that accompany them.

For various reasons, be they physical injury or environmental conditions, many people are unable to find the right path to their capabilities. Of course, there might be cases where the tool functions normally expressed through the capabilities for loving and knowing are so blocked that the problem cannot be alleviated even after extensive treatment. But it is neither logical nor admissible to conclude that the basic capabilities are nonexistent simply because there is a disorder in the tool function and, hence, a seemingly hopeless prognosis. The hopelessness of the situation stems not just from the function of the disorder, but also from the historically determined cures that are available. A decision in the sense of a diagnostic judgement thus often requires that the therapist have the courage to step down from his objective pedestal and admit, "I can't help him yet" rather than conclude, "There's nothing that can be done for him."

From this point of view, neuroses and psychoses can represent imbalanced differentiations of the basic capabilities. The goal of the therapy is to put the existing barriers aside and open the way for integration by placing the person's ability to love in a position where it can support his ability for knowing, and vice versa.

On what basis are we to understand this danger, this threatened loss of unity? Man can be regarded as a system where various elements and components have definite functions with each other. If one component or functional connection is disturbed, the whole system is affected.

Unity includes the tendency of an organism to sustain itself. This is clear even in normal development and self-preservation. Hunger reveals a lack of nourishment, a lack that man also experiences on an emotional level. At this point, a search begins that ends only when food is found, the shortage is alleviated, and the person again feels his needs have been satisfied. If we apply this example to the psychic realm, we can see why both experiences and things not experienced can lead to mental and psychosomatic disorders.

An experienced event includes a person's confrontation with certain behavioral norms that seem especially important to his partner. A child's industriousness, for example, can be endowed with extraordinary importance; the parent might load the child down with a lot of tasks and see that he is kept busy all the time. But this can hamper the child's ability to exercise his fantasy and develop the friendships that would provide the experiences necessary for a child his age. Here both the experienced and the unexperienced events can be sources of conflict.

A partner also brings his spouse conflicts, difficulties, problems, and crises. But the spouse is also given the opportunity for further development and possible solutions to existing problems. The confrontation has validity in many realms of life: in the relationship between children and parents; in the relationship between the parents; in relationships to in-laws and other people. It is a mistake to see only suffering in suffering, only danger in conflict. Such a view produces misunderstandings that have serious consequences in child rearing and psychotherapy.

It is therefore not enough to just examine the "why" of a disorder, sorrow, or test. These cases remain unknown if the question "For what?" is not also posed. An inquiry into "What for?" means reintegration, the tendency toward unity and further development.

When they are understood as the loss of unity, illnesses and disorders are not meaningless. They have special meaning in that they help reestablish or further develop the unity in personality.

5. The Basic Capabilities in the Literature

I discovered the hypotheses of the basic capabilities already set forth in similar form in the Baha'i religion (cf. Peseschkian, 1977, pp. 103–16). Their principles are shown in many forms. Sigmund Freud uses the dichotomy of the pleasure principle and the reality principle. Guildord (1965) speaks of universal dispositions and character traits. Maslow (1973) uses the concept of the basic needs of human existence. Fromm (1974) makes a distinction between the instincts biologically peculiar to all men and the existential needs. Erikson (1971) uses the concept of "basic virtues," which he describes in sequence. These various concepts are derived from different scientific theories and cannot automatically be applied to each other. But if we disregard the differences in their theoretical connections, we find an image of man for which constructs can be advanced that correspond to the basic capabilities.

The concept of the capabilities is accompanied by some insecurity. Capabilities are not immediately observable or measurable. They can first be perceived only when they are expressed as accomplishments. Every person possesses these capabilities. Whether or not they take shape in the course of his development depends on the supportive or inhibiting conditions of his body, his environment, and the times he lives in. These capabilities are part of the person's positive existence. They are really present, even if we do not see them at the moment. In this sense, the positive process means that we accept ourselves and our fellowmen as they are at the present time. But at the same time, we must also see what they can become. This requires that we first accept the person with his disorders and illnesses so that we can then establish contact with his capabilities that are yet unkown, hidden, and disturbed by his illness. The model for this process is the early relationship between parents and child. The child's capabilities clamor for outward expression. The related person—the mother, for instance—automatically develops in the child-rearing situation a relationship with capabilities that are still undeveloped and hence unknown to her. Although she cannot see the child's capabilities, she believes in their existence. This attitude toward the unknown makes it easier for her to put up with the child's clumsiness, his lack of hygiene, his impatient crying, et cetera. The child is toothless, can't walk, and can't speak, and yet the parents act as if he will master all these things in due time. The child's development and the parents' attitudes toward him can be transferred to the general problems of interpersonal relationships. But here again, it is not just a matter of focusing on shortcomings, difficulties, problems, disorders, and illnesses, but on the existing capabilities that enable us to deal with the disorders.

Whenever possible, we try to look at the total picture, at all the givens, not just the critical areas. Through this point of view we are able to dispel the image of the suffering, passive patient and understand him as the subject of self-help.

6. Possibilities for Reinterpretation

First learn, then teach.

—Oriental wisdom

In applied family therapy, the positive process means that we look for an encompassing overview of the capabilities of the family members so that we can develop interpretative possibilities for the behavior, symptom, or illness. This reevaluation paves the way for new therapeutic approaches. In terms of methodology, we draw primarily on transcultural-historical and metatheoretical reinterpretations.

TRANSCULTURAL REINTERPRETATION

In its German usage, the term "loneliness" has a positive connotation. In *William Tell,* Schiller wrote: "The strong person is mightiest when he is alone." As in this motto, many people believe that the ability to be independent and self-reliant is the epitome of strength. In Europe, it does not seem unusual if someone goes walking by himself so he can be alone with his thoughts. But in the Middle East, this kind of behavior arouses suspicion: "Is he insulted? Is he depressed or melancholy? It's not right for him or us that he isolates himself this way. If he's got a problem, we can help him!" The attempt to be alone and to withdraw from social contact is interpreted as a disorder within the mutual trust. These differing views of the same behavior produce different reactions from people of different cultures and reflect the different social rules operating in the different groups. They describe what is "normal"; they tell us when the border between the normal and the abnormal/sickly has been crossed. By realizing that the same behavior is measured by different standards in different cultures or epochs, a person finds that his horizons have expanded. He no longer measures behavior by proscribed criteria, but compares them with various views. This also has consequences for his interpersonal relationships. Through the relativization of his own value system, prejudices are questioned, fixations are overcome, and blocks to communication are lifted. All of these ideas correspond to one of the therapeutic principles of Positive Family Therapy: We are less likely to interpret a conspicuous behavioral pattern than we are to inquire about the game rules that cause the behavior to seem so conspicuous. We do this by enrichening the therapeutic, familiar system with views, concepts, and game rules from other cultures.

METATHEORETICAL REINTERPRETATION

According to the medical mode, illness is objectively present and is ascertained on the basis of evidence. This objectivity is supported by the observation that illnesses follow a determined course and that there can be therapeutic intervention during this predictable course.

But this model leaves some questions unanswered. What happens before it develops into an illness with a predictable course? What are the causal and conditional prerequisites and the risk factors that increase a person's receptivity to the disease, i.e., lower his resistance? To what extent is the course of the illness influenced by the attitudes of the patient and the people around him?

The treatment itself—even if it takes place *lege artis*—depends in large part of the diagnostic and therapeutic model that the therapist brings to the patient. This, in turn, is determined by what the therapist learned in his training, by what therapeutic possibilities appear accessible in terms of the theory being used, and by the form of treatment the patient wants, as expressed in his selection of the therapist.

In internal medicine, anxiety is usually viewed as the accompanying symptom for other ailments, such as angina pectoris. For a surgeon, this is a factor that must be taken into consideration before an operation; it can be remedied by tablets or an injection. In psychiatry, anxiety is regarded as a reaction to a frightening situation, as neurotic anxiety, or as the accompanying symptom of a psychosis. The doctor can make use of available medicines designed to relieve the anxiety. Psychoanalysis views anxiety as the result of a conflict between suppressed drives, internalized demands, and the controlling egofunctions. In behavioral therapy, anxiety is an acquired reaction with vegetative participation that can be unlearned by processes based on learning theory. Although all these directions mean "anxiety," they given the concept different meanings in both clinical observation and theory and call for different measures to combat it. The more ambiguous the symptom, the more noticeable the effect.

THE POSITIVE SYMPTOM

Illness, as a diminishment of one's subjective sense of being able to work and enjoy life, is considered a negative condition, particularly in a society that uses achievement as its yardstick. Given this point of view, the question about the "positive" aspects of an illness is targeted at areas that are frequently ignored: the significance of the illness for the way the patient processes his experiences; its function within the family structure; its meaning as an indicator of an imbalanced living situation; and, finally, the increased attention that it brings to the patient. The positive alternatives are not labels that one simply attaches to the patient in place of the previous diagnosis. They are justified by the fact that they contain a "program" and reveal new ways of approaching a conflict (Haley, 1973). Along with opening up new game rules for interpersonal relationships, the reinterpretations influence the patient's and his family's attitudes toward the illness and in this way help diminish the sense of suffering. This happens particularly because the patient and his family are not a blank page as far as the illness is concerned. Rather, they have a prescientific notion of the illness that determines how they adapt to it.

With a positive interpretation, the therapist does not just address the illness alone, but also the subjective ideas about the illness as transmitted through the traditions of the family.

7. Practical Applications of the "Positive Interpretations"

When a man is able to insult with a smile, he is worthy to become a leader.

Nachman of Bratslav

In the sense of "Positive Interpretations," I do not want *depression* to be understood simply as "the feeling of being depressed, with predominantly passive attitude." It also reflects the *ability to react with deep emotionalism. Fear of loneliness is not just the inability to get along on one's own; it also represents a strongly expressed need to develop relationships with other people.* An example of these positive interpretations can be found in the following dialogue with a thirty-two–year–old married woman, a patient suffering from severe depression.

Patient: *I feel like I'm a human wreck. . . . I'm so depressed and sad and sometimes have the feeling that it would be better if I could leave this world. [Patient begins to cry.] I feel so alone. No one has time for me. My husband lives only for his career. I always dread those lonely evenings when I wait for my husband and don't know when he'll come. . . .*

Therapist: *I have the impression you like to spend time with your husband and that you would also like to socialize more with other people.*

Patient: *I'd like to, but my husband doesn't have any time for such things. And I can't do them alone because he never says for sure when he'll come. . . .*

The patient is not led to repeatedly talk about her seemingly insolvable conflict. Instead, the therapist's comment (For example, "You like to be with your husband and with other people") put her problem in a new light. They created an impetus for her to seek new ways to deal with the problem and to distance herself from the old ideas she had talked about all too often.

Another example—important for educational counseling and the treatment of conflicts regarding career and employment—is centered on the issue of *laziness*. Laziness *is* conventionally defined as the lack of ambition. But there is something more to laziness—namely, the ability to avoid the demands for achievement. This positive interpretation becomes more important against the background of stress-related illnesses brought about by the demands of a career. Perhaps this definition also explains the aggressiveness with which industrious people react to the so-called loafers. Haley (1973) emphasizes the positive aspect from his point of view:

> *The experienced family therapist does not consider the idea of confronting family members with the fact that they hate each other. Instead of taking that approach, he is more inclined to interpret destructive behavior in a positive way, for instance as a protective treatment. . . . A newcomer to family therapy, for example, working with the family of a schizophrenic boy, observes how the mother petted her son on his backside. The therapist thought he was helping her by interpreting her behavior as the result of incestuous desires. But he merely succeeded in driving the mother and son even farther apart than before. An experienced therapist would have probably congratulated the mother for being able to use this gesture as a sign of her love for her child.*

A good example of the significance of a positive reinterpretation is provided by a fifty-six–year–old woman suffering from asthma. For eight years, she had been receiving somatic treatment, but without any success. During this time, she had been examined and treated in fourteen different clinics. Her situation and her asthma attacks were, in certain respects, very typical. She took care of her old mother with great dedication and saw to her every need, even though she felt that this was unfair and continually had to suppress her aggression and desires to be rid of this task. Furthermore, she felt overburdened at her job. Often she felt she had more than enough to do in taking care of her mother, let alone meeting the demands of her job. It finally came to the point that her family doctor advised her to apply for aid from the government.

I first met her when she was in this situation. The crucial task was to win her over to psychotherapy. In the sense of the positive process, I asked her what her asthma meant to her and, along with that, what positive aspects the illness offered her. She thought about this question over the course of several sessions. Without feeling insulted, she herself revealed the secondary benefits of the illness and recognized her asthma as a meaningful reaction to the excessive burdens she had at home and at work.

She wrote, among other things: "My asthma attacks demanded I call in sick. I simply longed for some peace and quiet and some respite from all the stress. . . ." The positive process opened the way for us to work on the conflict themes that played a role in her situation. In the third part of the treatment, the patient became a therapist for her mother, a function that allowed her to free herself from her infantile dependence and to develop a new definition of their relationship.

The positive reinterpretation of the illness was thus a starting point for the eventually successful treatment of two patients. These examples show how important a change of perspective can be in finding new solutions and, hence, new ways for self-help. This rethinking can be applied to almost all conflicts. If it doesn't immediately lead to dramatic improvement, it can at least produce a more distanced and differentiated relationship to the conflict. This can then become the starting point for an appropriate solution.

In this sense, every symptom and every illness can basically be interpreted in new ways. The rethinking deals less with the objective evidence than with the subjective processing of the disorder, which, again, will vary from group to group. Since symptoms are generally interpreted negatively, i.e., as insolvable and unpleasant, the positive interpretation fulfills a real need. Its goal is to produce a change in the understanding of an individual, family, or group so that new alternatives can be tried. In practice, it looks as if we inquire about the meaning a symptom has for a person and his group. We thus get at its "positive" meaning; "What are the positive aspects of blushing?" "What advantages do I get from my inhibitions?" "What functions are fulfilled by insomnia and other sleep disorders?" "What is meant by the fact that I have anxieties?"

This way of thinking, of course, is unusual for most people, for they associate disorders in their health and well-being with traditional—usually negatively colored—ideas. Positive reinterpretations are thus basically a stimulus for rethinking old concepts and for seeing if there aren't alternative interpretations and forms of treatment available for the patient.

We see our main task in enabling the patients to develop alternative attitudes to their illnesses and in appealing to therapists to be as flexible as possible in their treatments.

Examples of Change in Perspective

Traditional Interpretation	*Positive Interpretation*
Anorexia Nervosa	
Loss of appetite, slenderness mania at puberty.	The ability to get along with limited means. The ability to get out of the female sexual role through hunger. The ability to partake of the hunger of the world.
Alcoholism	
Dipsomania, psychological symptoms: euphoria (well-being), overestimation of oneself, loss of inhibitions, unrestrained conduct, tactlessness, obtrusiveness, loud behavior, tendency to react without reflection (transit violations and criminality).	The capacity to make conflicts temporarily bearable through the help of alcohol. The capacity to generate an illusion of protection based on the feeling of inner warmth, and through the loosening of inhibitions and anxieties to make it easier to accept one's own personality.
Ambivalent Attitude	
Ambivalence. Existence side by side of contradictory feelings in relation to the same object, e.g., love and hate at the same time. Erotic attachments and the relationship between parents and children are often markedly ambivalent.	The capacity not to become set in one's ways. *Capable of being enlarged upon:* the insight that one always runs a risk, dares to step into the unknown, carries the burden of doubt on one's shoulders, but still lives always with the hope of discovering a new capacity or a new frontier somewhere.

Traditional Interpretation	*Positive Interpretation*
Disobedience, Insolence	
Psychological rejection of outside authorities, often combined with emotional outbreaks (rage) (insolent phase).	The ability to say no. *Capable of being enlarged upon:* Time (when to say no), trust, reason (to learn when one should do something, or clarify why one says no).
Bedwetting	
Bedwetting is a special form of uncontrolled emptying of the bladder. It occurs at night, when one is lying in bed asleep.	The ability to recover earlier, not forgotten ways of reacting, when faced with difficult situations. The ability to cry downwards.
Depression	
The feeling of being despondent, with a prevailing passive attitude. Spiritual dejection, exhaustion.	The ability to react to conflicts with deep emotion. *Capable of being enlarged upon:* Relationship to the Thou, to the We, to the Origin-We, time, trust and hope.
Jealousy	
Rabid fear of losing a partner, coupled with inadequate control of reality. Intense abhorrence of a very possible rival, resulting from the claim to exclusiveness, especially in love.	The ability to love without behaving in such a way as to be loved. Positive relationship toward the I, toward the partner and toward faithfulness, pronounced fantasy. The ability to love one's partner and to attach oneself to him or her is stressed.

Existential Anxiety

Traditional Interpretation	*Positive Interpretation*
Insecurity, fear of the future, combined with psycho-vegetative disturbances.	The ability to provide for the future and not give in to the illusion of security. *Capable of being enlarged upon:* Differentiated relationship to the future, rationalization of the secondary capacities involved.

Fear of Attachment

Traditional Interpretation	*Positive Interpretation*
Defensive and ambivalent attitude of rejection of other people, social distance. Main symptom: inhibitions and feelings of depression, with some strong affective sharing.	Stress on the relationship to the I or to the existing partners. *Capable of being enlarged upon:* Contact, relationship to the We, courtesy, honesty, verbalization and broadening of goals.

Fear of Groups

Traditional Interpretation	*Positive Interpretation*
Defensive and ambivalent attitude of rejection of other people, social distance. Main symptom: inhibitions and feelings of depression, with some strong affective sharing.	Stress on the relationship to the I or to the existing partners. *Capable of being enlarged upon:* Contact, relationship to the We, courtesy, honesty, verbalization and broadening of goals.

Bronchial Asthma

Traditional Interpretation	*Positive Interpretation*
Fits of shortness of breath, through cramps in the bronchial muscles and, reflexively, in the diaphragm, as well as conditioned by the respiratory muscles.	Intensive relationship to one's own body, to a reference person; the ability to become aware of oneself through the symptom (rasping, coughing, gasping for breath). *Capable of being enlarged upon:* verbalizing conflicts (reason), attachment-detachment, honesty, trust, reliance, hope.

Traditional Interpretation	*Positive Interpretation*
Precocious Ejaculation	
Premature discharge of semen	The ability to reach one's goal quickly. Positive relationship to the partner, marked imprinting of diligence/achievement, time. *Capable of being enlarged upon:* time, patience, punctuality, reliability.
Laziness	
Inhibition of achievement, desertion, Lack of diligence, character weakness.	The ability to avoid achievement demands. *Capable of being enlarged upon:* Time (when and where one is lazy), differentiating and becoming aware of one's own capacities.
Fixation	
According to Freud, the persistence of drive activity at an earlier stage of development, in order to make it possible to hold on to childish ways of gaining satisfaction. Frequently fixation is directly connected to perversion and neurosis.	The ability to hold on to something. The ability to hold to attitudes and conduct. *Capable of being enlarged upon:* Every behavior and every attitude exists within the framework of some basic concept. The question is: when and under what circumstances does the fixation become a source of conflict?
Heart Attack	
Collapse of the tissues of the musculature of the heart, as a consequence of the closing of arteries around the heart.	The ability to take burdens and risk factors to heart. *Capable of being enlarged upon:* Correction of the achievement concept, change in eating habits (way of the senses), proper nutrition (way of reason) and building up of the relationship to the I, to one's own body.

Traditional Interpretation	*Positive Interpretation*
Compulsive Neurosis	
For example, repeatedly looking back to see if doors are closed, compulsive washing, compulsive ceremonies, the compulsion to go over the events of the day again and again in thought.	The ability to carry something through with extraordinary precision, conscientiousness, punctuality and consistency. The ability to mistrust oneself and, through repetition and controls, to ward off dangers: external dangers consciously, inner dangers unconsciously. Especially pronounced is the need for orderliness and reliability. *Capable of being enlarged upon:* certitude, time, contact, hope, future, the ability to let oneself be surprised.
Aggressivity	
Belligerence, brutality.	The ability to react spontaneously, emotionally and uninhibitedly to something. *Capable of being enlarged upon:* Against whom, when, where and in which form does aggression occur?
Frigidity	
The expression is derived from the Latin (frigidus—cold) and means sexual coldness and inability to have an orgasm on the part of women.	The ability to say no with the body. *Capable of being enlarged upon:* To develop the ability to also say no verbally. To better formulate one's own needs.

Traditional Interpretation	*Positive Interpretation*
Hypochondria	
Deep spiritual despondence by reason of imagined or insignificant physical ailments.	The ability to precisely observe one's own bodily functions and to perceive the organs' susceptibility to breakdown.
Criminality	
Committing of offenses punishable by law.	The ability to disregard rules of behavior. Positive relationship to the I, to a determined Thou or to a restricted We. *Capable of being enlarged upon:* Relationship to the We, Origin—We, thrift, justice, love, honesty, differentiated relationship to the near and distant future, taking into account the consequences.
Paranoia	
Madness, insanity, mental illness with primary crazy notions (delusions of persecution, grandeur, etc.).	The ability to see oneself as the mid-point of the world and its secret powers. *Capable of being enlarged upon:* Relationship to the other actual capacities, fantasy, reason, way of the senses, courtesy, honesty, trust and hope.
Phobia	
Fear of certain objects, such as mice, dogs, spiders, etc.; or of situations, e.g., fear of open spaces, closed areas or fear of blushing. On other occasions incipient hallucinations with feelings of anxiety.	The ability to avoid situations and objects which are experienced as threatening. *Capable of being enlarged upon:* The relationship to these situations and objects, contact, relationship to the I, Thou, We, Origin—We. Trust in the actual capacities involved at the moment.

Psychosomatic Symptoms

The triggering of physical signs of illness through psychological causes.

The ability to indicate through body language that at the time there is no other way of coping with conflict available.
Capable of being enlarged upon: Achievement, contact and future.

Masturbation

Sexual self satisfaction, onanism. This is a normal phase of sexual development (puberty), especially with the man, but should be considered abnormal if also continued when there is ample opportunity for sexual intercourse.

There exists an ability establish a relationship with one's own sexual parts.
Capable of being enlarged upon: The relationship to the Thou, to the relation with the partner (sexuality), interpersonal contact, honesty and cleanliness.

Narcissism

Way of being in love with one's own I, liking oneself.

The ability to love oneself and to experience one's own supposed weaknesses as positive.

Rivalry (Sibling Rivalry)

Jealous and tense relationship among siblings, inadequate readiness to show consideration.

The ability to affirm oneself through comparisons and to further develop.
Capable of being enlarged upon: Justice and love, uniqueness, contact, courtesy, honesty.

Sadism

Sexual arousal through inflicting pain, abusing, humiliating or soil-

The ability to take over the active role. The ability to enjoy the coning the loved one. Its most extreme expression is passion killing.

sciousness of one's own power and force.
Capable of being enlarged upon: Recognition of basic human capacities, justice, relationship to the We and the Origin—We.

Self-Neglect

External neglect—clothing, manners—should be distinguished from inward neglect of proper customs and morals.

The ability to ignore binding norms or to go against them.
Capable of being enlarged upon: Relationship to the I, to the Thou, the individual actual capacities (orderliness, honesty, courtesy, cleanliness, thrift, punctuality, etc.), paying attention to the development of trust and hope, attachment—discrimination and detachment.

Schizophrenia

The symptoms of schizophrenic psychosis are usually described in psychiatry in the following ways: absentmindedness, eccentricity, affectation, confused speech, stilted speech, stereotypes, desolation, et cetera. The behavior of the person is characterized as inadequate, bizarre, sloppy, cold, rigid, indecisive, indifferent, et cetera. Pseudophilosophic ideas, feigned depth, lack of affective resonance, neglect, and social isolation are listed as further traits. The ill persons are looked on as failures, as burdens to their families.

In former times and sometimes even today, the schizophrenic was claimed to have special capabilities. The pathos, the elevated speech, and the pensiveness of the patient were admired. According to Prinzhorn (1922), the schizophrenic is filled with a desire for the absolute. Jaspers (1948) attributed to them a sublime understanding and spiritual revelations. Mette (1928) found an increase in capabilities among them. He found an urge for extreme adequacy of expression, a need for direct reflection of feeling, a limitation to the most simple means of expression, a strong sensitivity to other people and things, an unusual neutrality regarding oneself, a particular refinement and intuition in psychological deductions, a richness of language in unusual images, and an elevated power of expressiveness. In family therapy, we have found that schizophrenics show a finer sensitivity to conflict, while their family members often appear to be indolent in relation to them. In its paranoid form, emphasis on fantasy and tradition (e.g., delusions of justice, religion, fidelity, politeness, et cetera). With hebephrenic forms, the ability to withdraw from areas of demands for achievement (actual capabilities) and to question these demands is present. With catatonics, motor withdrawal or its reverse, expression of excitement through uncoordinated movement is present. For those whose condition can be improved, to which contents is the delusion related? Which actual capabilities are still relatively stable (DAI)? To what media are the symptoms associated? Before pronouncing a judgment of "innate" or "indigenous," one should find out what has been done with the patient until now. Involve the family and social milieu as therapists. Psychiatric hospitals, which now function to some extent only as baby-sitting centers, should be changed into counseling offices, therapy centers, and outpatient clinics where the patients and their families can be prepared to participate in the therapeutic function.

Positive aspects of loneliness

A 37-year-old patient first began to change her life plans at the moment when she was able to grasp the positive aspects of her fate. Frequent stays at child care clinics due to bouts with asthma and developmental disturbances had set the trend for the development of her personality. The problem had been dealt with in previous psychotherapeutic treatment, in connection with fear of separation, the problem of leaving her parents and the syndrome of loneliness.

In the family in which she grew up it had been customary to talk a lot about the problem. Quite often she had been the center of attention: she was pitied either because of the problems that she had with her teacher or her father, or because of the problems she made for her family at mealtime. At the same time, she had learned that this talking about the problem made her the center of attention, while as the oldest child she would otherwise probably have received less attention. When she was ten years old, she stopped eating. Perhaps she unconsciously wanted to find out who in the family would stick with her and not let her die, and at the same time to provoke her father to show some concern for her.

Thus, through intensive involvement with problem situations she was prepared in a practical way for her choice of profession, which she herself later made, namely to become a social worker, and finally an educator, in order to be able to deal professionally with problems. Based on this emotional, intellectual and practical schooling during her childhood in recognizing problem situations, she can easily deal with many people's problems and difficulties, often perceiving things much sooner than her colleagues.

She made the following list of the positive effects of the stay at the child care clinics and of her problem:

- Through the experience of solitude and loneliness I better understand other people and their problems.
- Through this I can, in my opinion, better exercise my profession, have greater understanding and can offer advice.
- Good, friendly, deferential behavior toward my father's customers was positively received by my parents and by the customers, I was praised.
- Through this, I probably feel better in contact with others, avoiding criticism and keeping quiet about my own needs.
- I seldom approach other people, but rather wait for them to take the initiative—in this way I avoid the risk of being rejected, and thus escape being needlessly hurt and rejected.

- When I invite someone over, I prepare myself for it, thus winning the compliment that it is beautiful and cozy and that the food is delicious.
- I almost never spontaneously invite someone, in order to avoid disappointing the people, finding it boring or having the spontaneous joy taken away if I am refused.
- When before I gave up my desire to play and helped my mother around the house, she praised me.
- When I relinquished my desire to dance or go to parties or meet children of my own age, I was for the first time given preference over my sister; he praised me, saying that I was smart—I had waited for such recognition for years.
- As my mother often said she was afraid something might happen to me when I stayed away a long time, I wanted to avoid this reproach and make her happy, so more and more I relinquished contacts.
- Before I could never invite children of my own age, because we lived in crowded conditions, and besides I was ashamed of our apartment.
- When before I visited other children to play, I was able to escape from these narrow home behaviors and avoid the family's constant control, I felt freer.
- When later I more and more gave up playing and instead did my homework, I was recognized by my teachers as a diligent student and got good grades. This recognition was purchased at the cost of renunciation, but for me the attention, praise and recognition were vital.
- Today, by giving preference to contact with men who are educationally inferior to me, I avoid the risk of having to face intellectual exchanges, in which I am inevitably seen as inferior or dumb (I come from a working class family, where not much was read or discussed).
- Making contact spontaneously with many people, like my father did, was condemned by my mother and grandparents. I took that as an example to follow and completely avoided going to bars. Thus, when I relinquished spontaneous contact, I avoided being ignored or judged by the family.

The positive reinterpretation of the illness was thus a starting point for successful treatment. These examples show how important a change of perspective is for finding new possibilities for solution and, with these, self help.

Consequences

These translations are only examples and models for all other possible translations of illnesses and disturbances. The procedure is doubtless unusual for most people, for whom illnesses and disturbances are almost necessarily bound up with a negative or pessimistic concept. Such a concept is no guarantee of a more realistic view of things, but it can clarify why the reality of health and of psychiatric-psychotherapeutic care offers sufficient grounds for pessimism. When one loses sight of the positive aspects of an illness, one shouldn't be surprised at the consequences: that parents prematurely drive their children out of the house; that youth don't want to have anything more to do with their parents and with grown-ups; that marital partners separate or get divorced; that very many people retire early from their professions; that more and more people seek solutions to their problems in alcohol and in drugs; that people try to help others, without their actually being helped (as the example of developmental help shows); that people and groups hate one another, living side by side instead of working together for a better life for all; that the psychosomatically ill are thought to be simulating or are treated exclusively with medicaments; that mentally ill people are pushed over into abnormality; that psychiatric patients in clinics have to experience only custody, instead of psychotherapeutic treatment.

8. Aids for Changing One's Perspective

Why did God create but one man? So that no one of his descendants should be able to say, "My father is better than your father"?

—Talmud

One way of mobilizing the patients' resources instead of constantly rehashing old, familiar problems is for the therapist to provide stories and proverbs as counterconcepts.

By using stories, one can avoid the old one-way communication between therapist and patient. The therapist is no longer the one who, simply by virtue of his position, has all the answers and interpretations. Instead, there is a real exchange of concepts and counterconcepts. This requires a change of perspective on the part of the therapist and the patient so that both can learn from one another. When the gap between them is breached, the transition from psychotherapy to self-help becomes possible.

Many stories, parables, allegories, and proverbs make it easier to adopt an intellectual and emotional change of perspective. They accomplish this through their image-laden language, which stimulates not just logical thought, but also fantasy, intuition, and creativity. Furthermore, they serve as models and thus enable the listener to identify with the "hero" and thereby try out new solutions in his imagination. In child rearing, self-help and "folk therapy" stories have always occupied an important place. But even in the framework of critical self-help and modern psychotherapy they can provide the individual with important stimuli (Peseschkian, 1979).

A fifty-two–year–old woman experienced great anxieties when she had to be separated from her adult son. She complained that she had lost the ground under her feet: "Sometimes I'm overcome by the feeling that I've lived in vain. This happens when I think about my current situation. What have I accomplished in my life, and what do I really mean to my son? He hardly ever shows his face around here." At this

point, the concept of the woman clearly emerged: "Since I don't have my son [children] around here anymore, my life is meaningless. I am worthless."
To counter this idea, I told the patient a parable:

THE SECRET OF THE SEED

A seed offers itself for the tree that grows from it. Seen externally, the seed is lost, but the same seed that is sacrificed is embodied in the tree, its branches, blossoms, and fruits. If the continued existence of that seed had not been sacrificed for the tree, no branches, blossoms, or fruits could have developed.

—after Abdu'l'Bahá

The patient accepted this mythology as flattery, as an honor bestowed on her for her conduct. She was the one who had sacrificed herself, renounced her own interests, and finally achieved her son's being able to lead an independent and happy life. It did the patient good that her achievement was recognized. Only after her personal accomplishment was confirmed and she could feel secure in this recognition was she finally in a position to give up, step by step, her fixation with her singular and dominant reason for living—namely, her son.

This dissolution was no longer just a negative process for her, a contradiction of the maternal role. It was a step on the way to new interests and new goals.

9. What Are "Concepts"?

The man who accepts tradition without examining it with his own intelligence and judgment is like a blind man led by others.

—Bahya Ibn Paquda, *Duties of the Heart*

A central idea in positive family therapy is that of the *concept.* Psychology understands the term in the sense of a self-concept or an alient concept, hence as an image man has of himself or others. Concepts are thus cognitive and emotional structures that offer us the interpretive model for our relationships to ourselves, other people, and our environment. Contained in the concepts are the expectations that give our perceptions their unique color: whether we approach a partner pessimistically, critically, and mistrustfully or seek contact with him in an open, optimistic, and receptive manner. Here the behavioral component of the concepts is revealed. Instead of being pure ideas, they rest on the triad of cognition, emotion, and behavior. Concepts can be the motives that guide our behavior, adopted norms and habits that give us our direction. Because of their function, we designate the concepts as helmsmen: they tell a person where it's an uphill battle, what's good, what's bad, and which behavioral possibilities he has at his disposal. Although there is, in theory, an endless number of concepts, in practice there are relatively few. Each person has his own "program" of concepts that are partially interrelated and harmonious but can also create dissonance. In terms of contents, the concepts are described by the basic capabilities and the actual capabilities; their relational qualities are described by the four areas for processing conflict, the four model dimensions, and the forms of interaction. Beyond the individual, they work as game rules accepted by the entire group. As game rules, a part of our concept program matches the concepts of the group in which we live. They thus function as connective points in interpersonal relationships. As rules and normative systems, they regulate the interactions within a society. In view of the concepts, the family is given a special role. In the family, typical concepts are passed on, are restructured in response to human interactions, and are then adopted by the developing personality as part of daily life. Each individual, like each family unit, has typical behavioral patterns that can be traced back to a definite concept program: going to bed on time, getting up at a predetermined time, eating with the family at a certain time, being punctual, meeting responsibilities on time, feeling uncomfortable when there is a danger of being late, getting upset when other people are late, et cetera.

Behind these behavioral patterns and emotional reactions there is a behavioral style that is both personal and in conformance with the group and the role. It contains, for example, a typical concept of punctuality that can create possible conflicts in the marriage, family, or career if, for instance, the partner develops a more relaxed attitude toward punctuality.

10. Positive Family Therapy Does Not Remove Anything

Don't be too sweet, lest you be eaten up; don't be too bitter, lest you be spewed out.

—Oriental wisdom

The illness orientation in medicine and traditional psychotherapy triggers resistance on the part of the patients. One expects the doctor to take something away: the appendix, a few ounces of blood, one's favorite food. Just as the individual resists these kinds of interventions, so the patients and their families defend themselves against therapeutic measures that threaten to upset the family's balance. This can be the case when one expects reprimands from the therapist, when old habits and roles are questioned, or when family values are passed over.

With our positive process, we practitioners of Positive Family Therapy "disappoint"—in the original meaning of the term—the image that the patient and the family have of therapists. We neither make prohibitions nor indicate that we plan to take something away. On the contrary, we accept the symptomatic behavior and try to make the patient aware of the positive aspects of the disorder. Because of this process, the patients are not forced to defend themselves against the "attacker therapist." Instead, the therapist appears as an ally and achieves with the patient what could not be accomplished if they were battling each other. This is particularly important for the large group of potential patients who have successfully avoided every type of therapy: those who deny conflict. Although they have a lot of conflicts, suffer from the consequences, and cause others to suffer as well, they are afraid to face them directly. This behavior is rooted in their life history and obeys concepts that forbid a confrontation with the conflict. The denial of conflict works as a stabilizing force. We first turn our attention to this characteristic but do not scold the patient for his lack of insight. We thereby present him with an acceptable offer: that he drop his defensive posture on a trial basis and—supported by the positive interpretation—attempt to solve the conflict.

We believe the patient has the capacity for the illness, the symptom, and health. The therapist lends him primary support to the patient's regnerative capabilities. The family can strengthen the susceptibility to the illness, but it can also mobilize its capacity for health. The goal of Positive Family Therapy is to support the family in this activity for self-help.

11. The Patient as Therapist

We fall down by ourselves, but it takes a friendly hand to lift us up.

We have already seen that the patient possesses essential capabilities for self-help. Furthermore, we have noticed again and again that an illness and its consequences run their course not just in the individual, but also in the system in which he lives. In this regard, the family occupies the foreground as the primary and most direct relational group. Since a symptom is the expression of existing conflicts with the partner, family, or social group, the conflict takes on a special meaning within the particular group (Framo, 1973; Richter, 1979). Anxiety and inhibitions in a young wife, for example, allow her husband to step forward as her protector and demonstrate his own strength and inner stability. The recognition this brings to her husband enables the wife to forget that she has bought it at a high price, that she has paid for it with her own anxieties and weaknesses. For the wife, the husband's role as protector does afford her protection and security, but it also produces dependence, the lack of self-reliance, and the continuation of her social fears and inhibitions. There develops an apparent balance, a mutual shoring up that is more easily questioned by the "inhibited" partner—the one considered the patient—than by the other partner, the helper who is equally trapped in the problem (Selvini Palazzoli et al., 1977). This key position occupied by the alleged patient makes it easier to take a self-willed but effective step to change the situation.

In Positive Family Therapy, the patient gives up his patient role and becomes "psychotherapist" for his environment, especially his partner in the conflict (cf. also Minuchini, 1978; Selvini Palazzoli et al., 1977; Stierlin et al., 1977). Positive Family Therapy is dedicated primarily to this change in roles and thereby encourages the patients to embark on a conscious path toward self-help.

12. The Positive Procedure in the Therapeutic Process

One day's happiness makes a man forget his misfortune, and one day's misfortune makes him forget his past happiness.
—Ben Sirach,

In the therapeutic situation, the positive process begins by looking at three aspects:

a) *Observation of the Patient's Family and the Symptoms.* This aspect allows for a diagnostic orientation based on these questions: Which personality and communication structures are present, and which differential diagnostic considerations are possible? What does the patient offer the therapist?
b) *Positive Interpretation of the Symptoms.* We know that observation and the findings and diagnostic measures derived from it are not objective. Instead, the diagnostic relational systems of the therapist, his personal impressions, and the evaluations of the patient are also influential factors. In contrast to somatic medicine, this subjectivity is the crux of the matter in psycho- and family therapy. When we try other possibilities for evaluation (reinterpretation, positive interpretation, change of perspective), we do not do so because these might be objective. We do it as a way to relativise our own relational systems as well as those of the patient and his family. And we also want to initiate alternative solutions. We move away from the original symptoms and enter the areas where the patient feels he is "positive," i.e., relatively free of symptoms, ego-strong, and resistant. Two aspects are involved in all this: the reinterpretation of the symptom and the attention paid to the patient's capabilities.
c) *Reevaluation of the "Patient."* The patient's role as his own therapist and the positive interpretation of the symptoms improve the patient's position within the family (Schindler, R., 1976). The family structure thus takes on new importance as other members of the family are given the opportunity to step forward as patients. In this way, the family mechanisms for "sharing the illness" are

revealed. It can thus be determined which family member ended up bearing the symptoms and how this happened.

POSITIVE PROCESSES IN THE TREATMENT OF SOMATIC ILLNESSES

The positive process can be useful in treating therapy-resistant symptoms and illnesses that are primarily of a physical nature. The process helps the patients and their families find new connections with the disorder and deal with it in new ways. The suffering is thereby diminished: the illness is easier to bear. And there can also be positive changes in one's attitude to necessary medical measures, such as a difficult treatment, a limited diet, prostheses, or a frightening operation.

Part V:

Conflict Contents and Conflict Dynamics

1. Four Forms of Dealing with Conflict and How They Work

AN EASY CURE

The nephew of the ruler Ghabus-Woschmgir was seriously ill. All the physicians in the land had already given up hope. Their medicines had been to no avail. Since there was nothing more that the doctors could do, the ruler agreed that Avicena, who was a young man of sixteen at the time, should take over the treatment. When Avicena entered the palace, all were amazed at his courage, for he was determined to help the ailing man, even though all the wise hakims in the land had admitted their helplessness.

Avicena saw the ailing man, a thin, pale young man, stretched out on his bed. The man gave no reply to questions about his medical condition, and his relatives reported that he had not uttered a word for some time. Avicena took the man's pulse and held his hand for a long time. Finally he raised his head thoughtfully and said, "This young man needs a different kind of treatment. To provide that, I need someone who really knows this city, someone who knows all its streets and alleys, all the houses, and all the people living in them." All the people were amazed and asked, "What does healing a sick man have to do with the alleys of our city?" But in spite of their doubts, they obeyed Avicena's command and sent for a man who, so it was said, knew the city like the palm of his hand. Avicena said to him, "Name all the sections of the town for me." At the same time, he again took the patient's pulse.

When a certain quarter of the city was mentioned, Avicena felt the man's pulse quicken. Then he asked for the names of all the streets in that quarter, until the sick man's pulse again quickened at the sound of a particular street name. Now Avicena asked for the names of the alleys that ran into that street. The man was naming them one by one, when suddenly the name of a small, little-known alley produced a much greater response in the ailing man. Pleased with this response, Avicena commanded, "Bring me a man who can name all the houses in this alley, along with the people living in them." When they brought such a man to

Avicena, he had him name all the houses, and the sick man's pulse rate revealed which one Avicena was after.

When the man came to the names of the people living in that house, he also mentioned the name of a young woman. Immediately the patient's pulse began to race. The observant Avicena commented, "Very good. Everything is clear. I now know the young man's illness, and the cure is very simple." He got up and spoke to the people, all of whom were staring at him in amazement. "This young man is suffering from lovesickness. This is the root of his physical ailment. He is in love with the girl whose name you just heard. Go get the girl and woo her as a bride."

The patient who had listened to Avicena's words with great attention and excitement, blushed with embarrassment and crawled under the covers. The ruler proclaimed the girl as his nephew's bride, and the young man recovered within the hour.

—after Mowlana, Persian poet

In order to understand human conflicts, we inquire about the contents carried out by them. In the psychosocial realm, these contents are not static, but develop their own dynamics. They are most clearly evident in our relationships with the people who are important to us: our parents, grandparents, siblings, spouses, children, and others. The arising conflicts are played out on many levels at the same time: in the way we deal with experiences and in our relationships with our partners, our family, and larger social groups. To do justice to these various aspects, the contents with which we describe such conflicts must appear in these relational levels.

We want to deal with the various possibilities for grasping these conflict contents. We want to show how they influence the conflict dynamic. Although these methods are not dependent on one particular therapeutic arrangement, their focus is found in family therapy.

Despite all cultural and social differences and the uniqueness of each individual, we can observe that all people rely on four methods for dealing with their conflicts. When we have a problem, feel upset, burdened, or misunderstood, live in constant tension, or see no meaning in our lives, we can express these difficulties in the following four ways. These four ways are also linked to our four ways for learning and knowing. They enable us to see how man perceives himself and his environment and in what way reality is tested:

1. Body (by means of the sense)
2. Achievement (by means of reason)
3. Contact (by means of tradition)
4. Fantasy (by means of intuition)

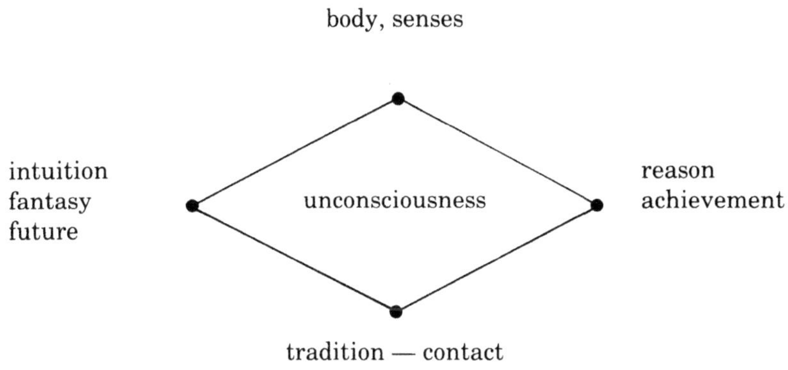

These forms for processing our conflicts are relatively broad categories that each person establishes with his own ideas, wishes, and conflicts.

Example: The father reacts by escaping into his work (achievement); the mother reacts by withdrawing, by avoiding social contact (contact); the child reacts with physical complaints (body). These various reactions can then lead to communication problems.

Each person develops his own preferences for dealing with problems that arise. Through hypertrophy of one way of dealing with conflict, the other forms fade into the background. The choice of one particular form depends to a great extent on the individual's learning experiences, especially ones stemming from childhood. The four forms of reaction are modelled in the concrete life situation as typical concepts.

QUESTIONS PROVIDING GENERAL ORIENTATION TO THE FOUR FORMS FOR DEALING WITH CONFLICT

1. How do you react when you have problems? (Do you respond with your body, through accomplishments, by looking to others for help, or in your fantasies?)
2. Which statement is true for you?: "I believe what I see." "I believe what I understand." "I believe what is transmitted to me—by my parents, for instance." "I believe what occurs to me spontaneously."
3. What was the motto at home? (For example, "food and drink keeps body and soul together"; "if you can do something, you are someone"; "What will people say?"; "God will take care of everything.")

APPLICATION OF THE FOUR FORMS FOR DEALING WITH CONFLICT

A patient said, "When I get upset, I get a headache that keeps me occupied for hours." We designate the answer this way:

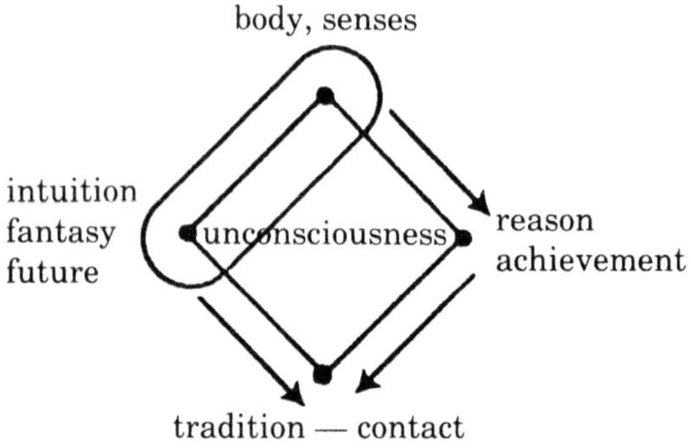

Dealing with Conflict: Body—Fantasy

To get further information, we asked, "How does your partner react to conflict?" The answer was "My husband retreats to his workroom in the basement and works like crazy almost all night. Sometimes I can hear him muttering out loud down there." The conflict areas are: "Industry/Achievement" and "Fantasy." It yielded this picture:

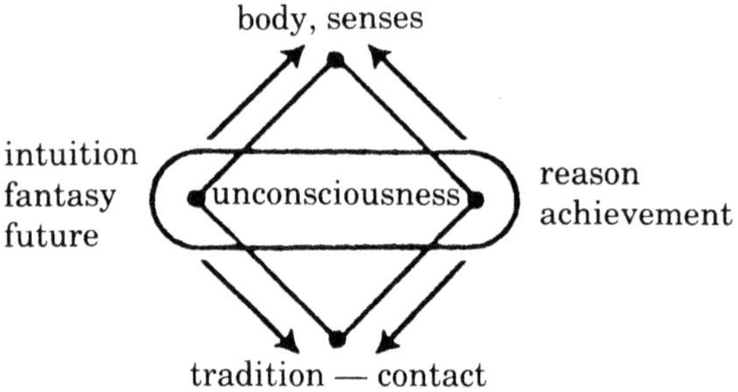

Dealing with Conflict: Achievement—Fantasy

In this way, we grasp individual reaction tendences and behavioral patterns as they occur more frequently in this partnership. A comparison of the two depictions shows that the body (neither partner has had much to say about sex for a long time) and contact remained uninvolved. In fact, further questioning reveals that contact is one area where there is a real deficiency in this marriage. But at first we disregard the conflictual area and deal with those things that seem most capable of development.

This procedure goes along with our positive point of view. A verbal image that I once used in connection with an achievement problem will illustrate how we proceed.

The four areas are like a rider who, motivated to achieve (Achievement) strives for a goal (Fantasy). To reach that goal, he needs a good horse that is well taken care of (Body); in case he gets thrown from the horse, he needs aides to help him get up again (Contact). This means the therapy cannot be concerned with just one area, e.g., the rider, but we must pay attention to all the areas involved.

In this way we can depict both individual styles for dealing with conflict and styles that are typical of a small group. Even reactions within an entire culture can be studied this way.

In my observations, I have found that in Europe and North America the areas "Body" and "Achievement" are generally in the foreground, whereas in the Mideast, there is a tendency to emphasize "Body," "Contact," and "Fantasy." Despite this tendency, each person experiences the world in his own way and develops a reaction pattern that matches his personality.

Somatically oriented physicians, for example, often have considerable trouble with patients from Southern Europe and the Mideast. These patients obviously have ailments, but the findings are not clear to the doctor. For this type of illness, the term "transalpine syndrome" has come to be used. Clues to the meaning of this syndrome, which appears in many forms, are found in the concepts determined by the patient's culture and family, on the one hand, and by the uprootedness and detachment of the foreign workers in Europe on the other.Since ties with the family organization have been lost, the person reacts to the conflict with his body.

The four areas for dealing with the conflict can help the therapist by pointing to major aspects of the disorder. Often these aspects are not seen by the machinery of organic-medical diagnoses and therapy.

BODY/SENSES

In the foreground stands the body-ego feeling. How does one perceive his body? How does one experience the various sensory impressions and the information coming from the environment? Information received through the senses is censored by acquired value standards. The individual sensory qualities can become conflict-laden in connection with the particular experiences. At the beginning of his development, a child establishes contact with the world through his senses. The totality of the activities is controlled by the senses.

Sleeping and feeding rhythms can be very important for the development of the child's punctuality. Some people panic when they hear someone crying. Memories of parents crying angrily or of the parents pleading that the children be quiet make noise subjectively unbearable. Other sensory qualities can also be affected. A dirty appearance alone is no cause for alarm. Only after we have learned on our own bodies that dirt is something bad and that being dirty is disgusting do we react so disgustedly when we see a filthy person. These areas thus become the site for diminished resistance and increased susceptibility. Conflicts are dealt with psychologically and psychosomatically.

We can better understand why a psychosomatic patient choses a particular organ if we examine the concepts he holds with regard to his body and to the individual organs and their functions. When a conflict occurs, the concepts determine why one man reacts with his heart, another with his stomach, another with his respiratory system, another with his skin, et cetera, and why some people escape into illness while others deny physical weakness and illness with all their might. Questions about these concepts can give the patient insight into his conflict and make him more amenable to psychotherapy. With a number of stomach patients, for example, as well as with obese persons, we discovered concepts related to nourishment ("what's brought to the table gets eaten"). On the other hand, we found that heart patients frequently had concepts related to promptness and the division of time. Rheumatic patients showed mostly typical problems with politeness ("Pull yourself together. What will people think?"). In patients with psychosomatic skin ailments, there were frequently conflict-laden concepts about cleanliness and contact.

Physical reactions to conflicts are: physical activity (involvement in sports or the opposite, taking things easy); sleep ("oversleep your conflicts"—sleep disorders); eating (gluttony, eating when you're unhappy, refusing to eat—anorexia nervosa); sex (playing Don Juan, nymphomania, aversion to sex), disorders in bodily functions and psychosomatic reactions. *Example:* "Every time I get upset because my husband is late, I get a headache."

Concepts such as "What's brought to the table gets eaten"; "One should torment his body so he doesn't lose his desire for death"; "You look pale, so you must be sick"; "Food and drink hold body and soul together"; et cetera can influence a person's attitudes to the body and to physical illnesses. They are one reason why people react to physical problems in such different ways—why some live like hypochondriacs, always expecting pain or illness, why others suppress their physical disorders.

Questions regarding the First Area for Dealing with Conflict

1. What physical complaints do you have? Which parts of the body are involved?
2. How do you judge your appearance?
3. Do you regard your body as friend or foe?
4. Is it important to you that your mate be good-looking?
5. Which of the five sense have the most meaning for you?
6. With which part of the body do you react when you are angry?
7. How does your mate (or family) react when you are sick?
8. How do you act when your mate is ill?
9. Do you need a lot of sleep or just a little?
10. How do illnesses affect your view of life and your attitudes about the future?
11. Does your family place a lot of importance on good appearance, athletic activities, and physical health?
12. When you were a child who in your family caressed, kissed, and was tender with you?
13. When you were a child was a lot of emphasis placed on good and abundant food in your home? What was the motto?
14. How did your parents react when you played with your body (e.g., thumb sucking, masturbation)?
15. How were you punished for playing with your body when you were a child (spanking, scolding, threats, hollering, withdrawal of food, withdrawal of love, et cetera)?
16. As a child, did you have to keep going to school even if you were sick?
17. As a child, did you have to go to bed immediately when you were sick?
18. When you were a child, who took care of you when you were sick?

ACHIEVEMENT (REASON)

This dimension is especially important in industrial society, particularly in the American-European cultural circle. It includes the way the norms of achievement are defined and incorporated into one's self-concept. Thought and reason make it possible to solve problems in a systematic, conscious way and to optimize achievement. Two opposing conflict reactions are possible: (a) escape into work and (b) escape from the demands of achievement. Typical symptoms are problems of self-worth, excessive demands, stress reactions, fear of failure, difficulty with concentration, and deficit symptoms like pension neuroses, apathy, fear of success, et cetera.

Concepts

"If you can do something, you are someone."
"First school, then play."
"Business is business and fun is fun."
"When you're learning you can't be the master."
"Time is money," et cetera.

Questions regarding the Second Area for Dealing with Conflict

1. What activities would you like to be doing? Are you satisfied with your career?
2. What activities are hard for you?
3. Is it important for you to always excel?
4. What are you most interested in (physical, intellectual, artistic activities, administrative tasks, et cetera)?
5. Is it easy for you to acknowledge the achievements of your spouse and children (e.g., do you dislike what he or she does, or does it bother you that he or she neglects you because of these activities)?
6. Do you consider yourself and your spouse to be intelligent?
7. When you assess a person, how important is his intelligence and social prestige?
8. Is it sometimes hard for you to make a decision?
9. What are you more involved in—your career or your family?

10. Do you feel comfortable when you don't have something to do?
11. Which of your parents placed more importance on achievement?
12. Which of your family members played with you when you were a child?
13. Who was most concerned about your homework when you were a child?
14. As a child, how were you punished when you made a mistake?
15. Did your parents tell you *why* you were supposed to do something when you were a child?
16. When you were a child, did your parents have an understanding of the things you were interested in?
17. Which experiences best typify your school years?
18. How were you rewarded for your accomplishments?

CONTACT (TRADITION)

This area comprises the ability to develop and maintain relationships: with oneself, one's mate, family, other people, groups, social classes, and foreign cultural circles, and animals, plants, and things. Patterns of social behavior are characterized by individual experiences and by tradition. Our possibilities for forming contacts and the socially acquired criteria that govern them are regulated: one expects his partner to show, e.g., politeness, honesty, justice, order, activity in certain areas of interest, et cetera and one seeks partners who match these criteria in some way.

We can react to conflicts by carrying the problem into our relationships with the environment. One extreme is the escape into sociability, whereby the protectiveness and activity of the group are supposed to help defuse the problem. By talking with other people, one tries to gain sympathy and solidarity: "When I'm upset about my mother-in-law, I usually call a girl friend and talk to her about it for hours on end." Here we find social hyperactivity, emotional dependence on groups, et cetera. But the reverse can also take place. One can withdraw from the group, distancing himself from the people who upset him. He feels inhibited and avoids social gatherings and other opportunities to get together with people. The symptoms are: inhibitions, unconscious need to cling to someone, fear of contact, prejudices, autism, et cetera.

Concepts

"What do I need other people for?"
"Man by himself is weak; when united with others, he is strong."
"Guests are a gift from God."
"You rely on yourself, but never on other people."
"A person without friends is only half a person."

Questions regarding the Third Area for Dealing with Conflict

1. Who in your family is more open to contacts?
2. Who in your family prefers to invite company to your house?
3. What would be more likely to prevent you from having company: the expense; the fact that guests might mess up the house; the fact that guests are a lot of work; the fact that you have to wait for some guests; your feeling that you can't offer your guests enough, et cetera?
4. How do you feel when you're with a lot of people at a party?
5. With which people is it hard for you to establish contact?
6. Which is easier for you, to establish contacts or to maintain them?
7. Is it hard for you to give up your favorite customs?
8. What does tradition mean to you?
9. Do you adhere to family (religious, political) traditions?
10. Are you particularly concerned about what other people could say?
11. Which of your parents was more sociable?
12. Did you have many friends when you were a child or were you more isolated?
13. When your parents had company, were you allowed to be present and participate?
14. As a child, to whom could you turn when you had problems?
15. Is contact with relatives important to you?
16. As a child, did you have a lot of playmates, or did you usually play alone?
17. When you were a child, did your parents place a lot of importance on good behavior and politeness?
18. What memories do you associate with these questions?

FANTASY (INTUITION)

A further means of awareness is what is poetically called the language of the heart or suggestion; in the language of religion, it is referred to as inspiration, and in psychology it is known as intuition or intuitive judgment. In this connection, intuition seems related to the psychic process of the dream or fantasy—processes that can also represent a way of dealing with problems and conflicts. One can react to conflicts by activating one's fantasy—by fantasizing about a solution, by imagining the desired results, by picturing that the antagonist is punished or even killed.

In creative actions and sexual fantasies, for example, fantasy and intuition can arouse needs and even satisfy them. As a "private world," fantasy shields one from dangerous and threatening intrusions by reality and thus creates a provisional comfortable sphere (e.g., in alcohol and drug abuse). Fantasy can make a "bad deed" and a painful separation from one's spouse seem unreal. But it can also cause anxiety and become overpowering. In this way, fantasy becomes confused with perceptions and leads to symptoms such as the illusions that occur in schizophrenia. In order to keep the frightening dynamic power of fantasy under control, some people adopt a compulsive kind of behavior; like a corset, it helps them keep their threatening fantasies in rein and protects them from uncontrollable outbreaks of emotion.

Intuition and fantasy go beyond the immediate reality and can encompass everything we describe as the meaning of activity, the meaning of life, desire, ideas about the future, and utopia. Philosophies and religions enter into the capacity for intuition-fantasy and thereby establish connections to a more distant future.

The essence of fantasy is the feeling of being drawn toward the unknown. The capacity for fantasy "is accompanied by the fact that one risks taking that step into the unknown, takes the burden of doubt on his shoulders and nevertheless lives in the hope of somewhere discovering a new capacity or a new limit (which is also a part of his own reality)" (Jordan, 1969). If there were no curiosity stemming from fantasy, there would be no doubt and no fear; but without doubt and fear, there would be no development, no progress, no self-discovery for man.

Man's longing for the unknown—we purposely formulate it in these vague terms because it can have a different shape for each person and each situation—has led to the fact that, throughout all of world history, this longing has spoken to the founders of religions.

Imaginary experimentation, fantasies accompanied by action, and fantasies that provide relief have taken on a traditional form in fairy tales, narratives, and stories. In the fairy tale, there is a meeting of transmitted fantasies and the fantasies of the individual person. Similar overlappings can be found in other artistic, creative, and productive activities. The acquired learnings in the other areas for processing conflict filter the formational possibilities of fantasy. An example of this is the lessening of playful fantasy in achievement-oriented people of modern industrial society.

The capacity for fantasy develops very early, at a time when the child cannot yet distinguish between reality and imagination and is unable to establish clear causal relationships. Fantasy develops through play. The course of this development is influenced by the way the family concepts include the readiness to deal with fantasy and its contents.

Concepts

"It's all in your imagination."
"Why should I care about reality as long as I'm happy?"
"Thank God death isn't the end of it all."
"He who dares, wins."
"Unhappy without a wish."
"In time, a solution will come."

Questions regarding the Fourth Area for Dealing with Conflicts

1. Who in your family places more importance on fantasy?
2. Do you often hit upon a good idea?
3. Do you sometimes prefer fantasy to reality?
4. What are your preoccupations in your fantasies: the body (sex, sleep, sports), career (success, failure), contact with other people, the future (wishes, philosophies, religion)?
5. Do you like to cling to the past?
6. Do you sometimes think about how your life would be with a different spouse, a different profession, et cetera?
7. Which characteristics of your spouse have the most significance in your fantasies?

8. Do you like to think about the future? Do you enjoy reading utopian literature?
9. Have you ever toyed with the idea of committing suicide?
10. If you could change places with someone for a week, who would you choose to be? Why?
11. If you were invisible for a day, how would you spend your time?
12. Who, if anyone, would you choose as your model?
13. Can you still remember fantasies you had as a child?
14. Which of your family members had more understanding of fantasies and daydreams?
15. With whom could (can) you best spin out your dreams?
16. What relationship do you have to art (painting, music, literature)? Do you paint? If so, what do your paintings express?
17. How do you visualize life after death?
18. Which memories occur to you in connection with these questions?

THE UNCONSCIOUS

Only a portion of the motives behind human behavior reach consciousness and are controlled by it. Freud's psychoanalysis is based on this realization. He formulated the theory of the unconscious, a theory in which the sexual life is given particular importance.

In Positive Family Therapy, the two basic capabilities of awareness and love replace the libido of Freudian theory. To a certain extent, the libido is rooted in the basic capabilities as an energetic component. In addition, the unconscious has the following two functions in Positive Family Therapy.

First, it is the site of the undeveloped, undifferentiated capabilities and human energy. Resting in the unconscious is everything that is inherent in man but not yet developed because the conditions for its maturation has not yet arrived. The capabilities are energy potentials that strive for realization.

Second, the unconscious is the site of suppressed and repressed actual capabilities and media. The individual capabilities have already undergone a confrontation with the environment; they have either been rejected by the environment, the environment has offered no significant conditions for their development, or other actual capabilities were given such emphasis that there was no place left for the remaining ones.

Against this background of the two-fold function of the unconscious, one can understand why experiences are not the sole causes of disorders and conflicts; one can see that things *not* experienced can also be a factor.

Because of its very nature, the unconscious is inaccessible to direct questioning. But it can be opened up by the therapist. In the therapeutic situation, the unconscious is less accessible than the contents that can be perceived and are thus labeled as preconscious.

The therapist tries to determine the psychodynamically effective connections based on the information at hand—the patterns of actual capabilities and the patient's ability to love and to understand. The concepts, derived from the person's life story, keep individual psychic contents separate from the conscious and remove them from its control. In view of the four areas for dealing with conflict, this process can be described as insufficient differentiation, as one-sidedness. When, for instance, the area "achievement/understanding" occupies the midpoint, it can mean that one's relationships to one's body and to other people (contact) are suppressed. Even fantasy is regulated by this imbalance. Individual dreams and fantasies likewise deal only with achievements. Similar mechanisms can be observed with regard to one's ability to love and, as we will see later on, with regard to the actual capabilities.

To be sure, man has potential access to all the possibilities for dealing with conflict, but his concepts allow him to take up only a few of them, thus blocking his access to the other forms for dealing with the conflicts. In large part, the therapeutic task involves making these concepts conscious and available. The therapist seeks to uncover the patients' psychodynamic backgrounds and provide easier access to the previously undifferentiated capabilities.

Working with the instruments of Positive Family Therapy is in this sense a way to open up the preconscious and the unconscious.

2. The Four Forms of Dealing with Conflict, as Used in Positive Family Therapy

There are three types of friends: those like food, without which you can't live; those like medicine, which you need occasionally; and those like an illness, which you never want.

—Ibn Gabirol

In terms of family therapy, the four areas for dealing with conflict have the following functions.

The media for learning and knowing represent tools that characterize the individual styles one adopts in order to deal with reality and conflict. Two forms can be differentiated:

a) Attitudes about the media in question—These attitudes help us determine the value the particular media hold within the patient's self-concept. They can be revealed by statements like "Why be cuddled, and why all these tender gestures? What counts with me is that I be successful and keep my wits about me" or "From everything I see and hear, I know that this man is married and doesn't love me at all. But I don't care. All I care about is the idea of his love."

b) Connecting points for the symptoms, which can be interpreted to some extent as disorders within the media for learning and knowing. We can thus include in the area "body senses" such symptoms as sleep disorders, loss of appetite, intestinal problems, irritability, compulsive eating, lack of exercise, visual and acoustical hallucinations, hypochondria, and disorders in one's perceptions, drives, and affects. Related to the area of "reason" are disorders in thought and intelligence; problems with concentration, memory, and decision making; the tendency to rationalize, to brood, to have compulsive thoughts, to lack connection with reality; et cetera. Fixations, prejudices, stereotypes, fanaticism, poor judgment, fear of the truth, hatred, narrow-mindedness, guilt, and lack of history are all associated with "tradition." Extreme fantasies, alienation from reality, suicide fantasies, sexual illusions, fears, compulsions, delusions, and paranoia can be included in the media of "fantasy—intuition."

Clues to the genesis of attitudes about these categories and their meaning within the symptoms can be acquired by examining the basic conflict.

Through the process, the family members are led to see the connections between the forms of dealing with conflict, the family concepts, and the symptoms. They gain insight into the particular style for responding to a conflict within a given social situation. This process reveals a segment of nonverbal communication that is included among the symptoms. In the family's everyday life, the chosen forms for dealing with conflict are an open secret: open because they are revealed to the partner by the individual's unique reactions, a secret because no one usually talks about them. This is why our process helps eliminate communication blocks within a family.

By inquiring about the areas for dealing with conflict, one approaches the history of individual concepts. These life experiences are not private property. Rather, they take shape within the family relationships. The definition of a person's own position and his particular historical condition within the family makes it easier to change his position. This, of course, facilitates mutual understanding. But questions of this type conceal a danger, which I should point out: This kind of interrogation can lead to a formal "checking off" of information, where more emphasis is placed on the system than on the family's relationships. More important than the mere accumulation of data is the opportunity for self-discovery, the array of thematic associations, and the possibilities for gaining access to the life story. These functions make it possible to deal with the questions in a flexible way and to adapt them to the needs of the therapist-patient relationship.

The concrete family situation makes the question about the four areas a highly explosive one. The existing problem takes on a "real" character merely because of the presence of the "perpetrator," the spouse, children, or parents. It is no longer a matter of "imaginary" parents, as is the problem of transference in psychoanalysis. Instead, the problems can be directed right at the person involved. This process becomes even more complex when members of several generations, perhaps including grandparents, are included in the therapy.

The family members involved are not divided up according to the forms for dealing with conflict, but according to the focuses and imbalances they have developed in the course of their individual and collective history. The social prestige granted to the seemingly healthy members of the family no longer exists. Even these "healthy ones" react to conflict, albeit in different ways that match their particular conditions. This makes it easier for everyone, not just those directly affected, to discuss the conflicts. All of this helps to foster mutual understanding.

When family conversations turn away from customary areas of the conflict and take up issues that had previously been avoided, there is usually some resistance. The shift from an achievement-oriented attitude is thus associated with the revision of a number of concepts and habits. Revising one's concepts is usually perceived as a painful process, one that often produces a lot of guilt. In other words, the change of perspective within the four forms of conflict reaction is not simply a cognitive process carried out by reason alone. On the contrary, it involves feelings to a great degree (affective and emotional), but at the same time represents potential change of deeply embedded behavior.

The shift from one area to another is much like moving from an old apartment to a newer, more beautiful one. Although it has its advantages, it also involves a lot of effort and expense; it requires that one leave one's old environment and establish contact with new surroundings, new people, and new developmental possibilities that one cannot yet control.

It is important to think carefully about these defensive attitudes, for they do not mean that someone doesn't *want* to change; they mean that the idea of changing one's perspective and revising one's concepts is already such a real possibility that the person feels he must resist it. This is why we protect the patient and enable him to develop a change of perspective step by step, using models of conflict reaction that he can control himself. By offering positive interpretations, the therapist supports the patient's family in its quest for new discoveries.

The four areas for dealing with conflict correspond to our ability to learn and to know, i.e., the means by which we come to terms with reality. Another essential dimension of human life is circumscribed by the ability to love, an ability that develops through our relationship with the environment. Because of this, we also investigate the quality of the relationship that can open the way for shaping our emotional selves.

3. The Four Model Dimensions

LATE REVENGE

A man was punished by his fellow villagers by being thrown into a dry cistern. The townspeople who had been treated unjustly by him took justice into their own hands. Some stood at the rim of the ditch and unleashed a shower of spit upon the man. Others threw mud from the street. Suddenly the man was hit by a stone. In amazement, he looked up and asked the stone thrower, "I know all the other people. Who are you, that you think you can throw stones at me?"

The man up on the edge of the ditch replied, "I'm the man you treated badly twenty years ago."

The sinner then asked, "Where were you all this time?"

"The whole time," the man answered, "I carried the stone in my heart. Now that I have found you in such a wretched condition, I took the stone in my hand."

The following model deals with the concepts that were valid in the original family group. In developing this model, we hold to two conditions: first, the concepts must have meaning for socialization; second, they must describe relationships to the environment. These concepts are transmitted by relatives such as parents, siblings, and grand*parents* or by people who have taken over these relatives' functions. The four model dimensions describe the pattern of family concepts in which the individual grows up in a way that reflects the individual's experience of them.

To understand the conflict, it is necessary to understand its background and the concepts involved. The development of the personality is stamped to a great degree by the person's primary social ties. We have found that it is worthwhile to use the model dimension to determine why a person prefers some relationships and rejects others. The relevant information deals with the following:

ties that the relational persons (parents) and siblings (or other playmates) have with the child ("I");

the relationship between the parents themselves ("you");
the parents' relationship to their environment ("we");
the parents' relationship to religion and their philosophy of life (Primal "We").

This model is also valid if the child grows up in an incomplete family or in an institution that substitutes for the family. In such a case, other people (grandparents, foster parents, or even teachers) represent the parents whose role they have more or less adopted. The stability that these relationships can develop is also included in the model.

The extent to which any of these four model dimensions is emphasized can vary with the individual. They are touched upon during the initial interview, but the problems they bring to light must be treated more extensively if and when therapy takes place later on.

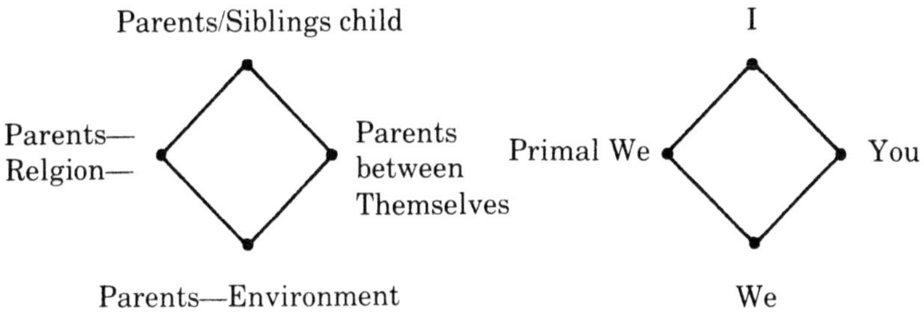

BASIS CONFLICT
(imprinting relationships)

ACTUAL CONFLICT
(structure of actual relationships)

The Model Dimension and the Development of the Four Media for the Ability of Loving

The four model dimensions, described as the basic conflict, are projected onto a person's relationships within the family and beyond it. The person incorporates both his experiences with the other people and the models they represent. These model relationships can be described separately as actual and basic conflicts, but in practice we project the two models onto each other and describe them as a common model.

The four model dimensions overlap with the four areas for dealing with conflict. In particular, there is correlation between the themes of "contact" and the relationship to "You—We" and between fantasy and the relationship to the "Primal 'We.'" Of course, one should avoid overlapping them during the investigation; a particular question should be given only as much weight as is called for by the situation.

The questions ask why the person has trouble accepting himself, why he tries to distance himself from his family, or why he is so tangled up in it; and what criteria he uses in developing relationships with his mate, other people, and groups. The agenda of questions also includes problems of social, racial, political, and religious prejudices. It is at this point that one can see why this procedure is important for a transcultural approach. It reveals various possibilities for dealing with people of various subcultures and national origins.

The four model dimensions are the possibilities every person has for developing relationships. They comprise the relationships to "I", "you" "we," and the "Primal We," which are discovered via the models from the original family.

Model means identification with a figure, the imitation of role aspects, the adoption of desired characteristics, and the cessation of undesirable ones. Aside from positive identification, there is also the possibility of using a "bad model" as a warning or as the stimulus to try other alternatives. One wants to avoid the mistakes of one's parents, for example. Many facets of a situation play a role in the formation of models: How do the parents view themselves and the image they want to present? How did the child perceive the parents and their behavior? To what extent is the parents' behavior harmonious; in what ways do they clash? Do the parents' concepts differ from those of other people in their surroundings? How would the individual resolve these differences? In other words, which model could he accept for himself?

In order to learn about the relationship between the parents and the child, we ask the person which parent had more time for him, which parent was more patient, and which parent he looked to as his model.

Relationships of parents and siblings to me

	Mother	Father
Time		
Patience		
Model		

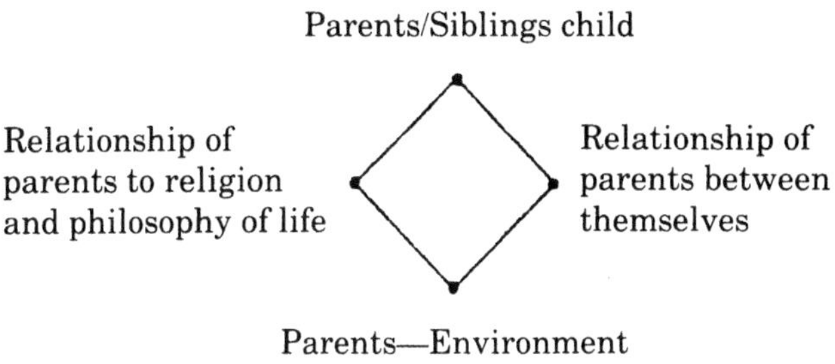

Schematic Overview of the Four Model Dimensions

For a quick overview of the evaluations of the four model dimensions, the reactions within each area are marked with a + or a − depending on their subjective quality. The differentiation of patience, time, and model is added alongside the four model dimensions. In family therapy, this process can be differentiated by adding the evaluations of other family members (father, mother, siblings, et cetera) in the same way. This notational system makes it easier to get a good overview of the situation and also serves the therapist as a memory aid. It also helps the family members get a better understanding of a situation by which they have felt overwhelmed.

INITIAL QUESTIONS

1. Who did you feel more closely tied to as a child (father, mother, grandparents)?
2. Which of your parents (or other significant persons) had more time for you?
3. Which parent was more patient, i.e., who was less likely to get upset?
4. Who was your model?
5. Do you feel you were treated fairly as a child? (Were your siblings, for instance, given preferential treatment?)
6. How do you assess your parents' marriage today?
7. Which parent was more open?
8. Which parent was more concerned with religious and philosophical questions?

RELATIONSHIP TO "I" (PARENTS/SIBLINGS—CHILD)

THE DIRTY NESTS

A dove was constantly changing her nest. The strong smell that the nests had developed over time was unbearable for her. She complained about this bitterly as she spoke with a wise, old, and experienced dove. The latter nodded his head several times and said, "By changing your nest all the time, you don't change anything. The smell that bothers you does not come from the nests but from you."

A person's relationship to himself depends particularly on how his desires and needs are satisfied. "Am I accepted or rejected?" This question finds its direct answer in the relationship between the child and the parent and later in comparison with the way the siblings are treated: "Whenever I messed up my room, I was always told how good my younger brother was. And that was always too much for me. My mother could get terribly upset if something wasn't in the right place. She would scold and then not talk with us for hours and even refuse to give us our allowance," says a twenty-eight–year–old female patient (mother of one child), who was referred for psychotherapeutic treatment because of frigidity and depression.

With socialization—the adoption of concepts and interpersonal game rules—another theme becomes important: "Am I accepted for myself or because of my accomplishments? "The child's perception of how his parents expend their time and patience is reflected in whom he chooses as his model. On this level, decisions are made according to basic emotional ties: original trust or mistrust, hope or desperation, positive or negative self-images. "I was particularly praised when I was clean and kept my clothes neat. Dirt was the worst thing that could happen to me." At this developmental level, the self-image and the body-I feeling (body/senses) are developed.

Concepts

"No one likes me, and I don't like myself either."
"I'm a lucky person."
"Everything I touch turns out well."
"I have faith in myself."
"I always need someone to help me."
"First me, then the others."

"I'm a failure."
"I'm just unlucky."
"Why bother? It won't do any good."

Questions regarding the First Model Dimension (Relationship to "I")

1. Who are you closer to (father, mother, grandparents)?
2. Who had more time for you when you were a child (father, mother, etc.)?
3. Which parent was more patient, i.e., who was less likely to get upset?
4. Who was your model? Whose behavior and attitudes have you adopted?
5. Do you feel you were treated fairly as a child? Were you or your siblings given preferential treatment?
6. How were you and your siblings punished?
7. How did your parents show their love to you (tenderness, warmth)?
8. Do you feel your parents wanted you?
9. How would you have had to develop to meet your parents' ideal?
10. Would your parents have preferred a boy or girl?

The questions regarding the area "body/senses" can complement the questions for the "relationship to 'I' ".

THE RELATIONSHIP TO "YOU" (PARENTS BETWEEN THEMSELVES)

FIFTY YEARS OF POLITNESS

An elderly couple celebrated their golden anniversary after long years of marriage. While eating breakfast together, the woman thought. For fifty years I've always been considerate of my husband and have always given him the crusty top of the breakfast roll. Today I want finally to enjoy this delicacy for myself. She spread the top part of the roll with butter and gave the other part to her husband. Contrary to her expectations, he was very pleased, kissed her hand, and said, "My darling, you've just given me the greatest joy of the day. For over fifty years I haven't eaten the bottom part of the roll, which is the part I like best. I always thought you should have it because you like it so much."

The relationship to "You" is already pre-formed through the experiences of the symbiotic mother-child relationship. The relationship to "I" that forms here is the initial stage of a differentiated relationship to one's partner. An emotional relationship like this, which can be described with terms like "affection," "love," and "community," marks the relationship to "You." The model for it is the example the parents' set in their relationship to each other. They exemplify definite forms of partnership that are peculiar to them. These become the standard for the child.

Concepts

The ideas one holds about partnership, marriage, community, sexuality, et cetera can be traced back in many respects to the model experiences, models, and concepts: "Someday, I'd like to have as harmonious a marriage as my parents' " or "I simply don't want to get married, have kids, and continue doing the same crap my grandparents and parents have done." Here there arises not only a general attitude about partnership and marriage but a number of behavioral patterns, ideas, and game rules: how the husband comes home; how his wife greets him; how the mother talks about him to the kids when he isn't around; how the family rituals surrounding eating, going to bed, recognizing personal accomplishments, and spending free time are dealt with in the family; how the parents show affection in public, particularly in front of the children (kisses, caresses, embraces, compliments); to what extent the parents discuss things that go beyond day-to-day topics and touch on themes like personal feelings, problems, desires, and goals; to what extent the parents effectively deal with conflicts or if they merely rebuke each other silently and hurt each other's feelings. The parents demonstrate their mutual dependencies and, along with them, their strategies for dealing with separation situations. The parents' conduct affects not just themselves but the entire family—indirectly in that the children adopt what they observe; directly when, for instance, the mother clings to the child when the father reveals that he wants to abandon the family.

The marriage's elasticity or brittleness—expressed by their partners' attitudes about fidelity—influences the concepts with regard to the exclusivity and duration of the relationship.

Questions regarding the Second Model Dimension (Relationship to "You")

1. Did your parents understand each other well?
2. Which parent had the most to say?
3. Did your parents form a united front in dealing with the children?
4. Do you think your parents married for love or for more practical reasons?
5. How did your parents deal with problems? (Were they able to speak openly with each other? Did they become violent? Did they dole out punishment by ignoring each other? Did they avoid conflicts by saying, "We don't have any problems"?)
6. Were your parents divorced or did the theme of separation appear in a different form?
7. Do you feel your parents treated you fairly?
8. What are your attitudes about partnership and marriage? What have been your experiences?
9. How do you feel about fidelity?
10. What ideas do you associate with partnership and the relationship to "You"? What situation came to mind as you answered these questions?

THE RELATIONSHIP TO "WE" (PARENTS—ENVIRONMENT)

GIVE HIM YOUR HAND

A man had sunk into a swamp in northern Persia. Only his head was still sticking out of the morass. At the top of his lungs, he screamed for help. Soon there gathered a crowd of people at the site of the accident. One decided to try to help the poor man. "Give me your hand," he cried over to him. "I will pull you out of the swamp." But the man stuck in the mud just kept crying for help and did nothing to enable the man to help him. "Give me your hand," the man demanded several times. But the answer was always just a wretched cry for help. Then someone else stepped up and said, "Don't you see that he will never give you his hand? You must give him your hand. Then you can save him."

The child's initial contacts with the outside world take place in his own way. He is curious, tries to grasp things around him, and overcomes his fear of people by virtue of his curiosity. At the same time, he becomes familiar with the way other family members shape their contacts outside the family. He learns to differentiate between friend and foe and adopts criteria for making these distinctions. For example, he learns to be loyal to his family and to unite with them against threats from other people. It is here that the relationship between the inner group and outer group is formed. It influences the family's communicative possibilities with regard to the outside world. They are reflected in one's readiness to accept or reject more distant relatives, strangers, other groups and families, and people of other races, nationalities, and social classes. In this respect, the parents are a model for outside contacts. They invite company over, accept invitatios, take part in social events, talk with old friends, establish contact with new ones, break off old relationships, and carry on discussions in the family and with strangers. But the parental model is not the only determinant for the relationship to the societal environment. Other groups that one has contact with in the course of his development influence his understanding of interpersonal relationships. This means that openness, receptivity, and the recognition of other people and their human worth can be furthered—or that prejudices, racial hatred, ethnic egotism, and narcissism can be intensified. It is here that typical models of interpersonal behavior develop—politically relevant behaviors that take shape in the formation of political parties and are guided by the dominant powers in a society. The role assignments in the family wield influence in the workplace and in the social dynamic. The son, for example, can take on the family task of becoming the social climber. He graduates from a good school and then chooses a career that brings him a lot of prestige. This occurs not just as the unfolding of his own capabilities, but also as a result of the role assignments and tasks that were delegated to him by parents and family.

Compared to Western society, the Mideast family comprises a much larger circle. It includes all sorts of relatives, family friends, and acquaintances. Because of the support provided by the many opportunities for transference, the family's broad safety net, and the family members' sense of duty to each other, they are able to intercept and counteract premature separation anxieties and mourning reactions.

Concepts

> "Guests are gifts from Godl"
> "Relatives are like shoes. The tighter they are, the more they pinch."

"Company costs money and messes up the house."
"The strong person is most powerful when he is alone."
"If we just hang together, it makes no difference if the rest of the world falls apart."
"You as a person are nothing; your people are everything."
"Don't play with children who always look dirty."
"We'll stay in our group, and the others can stay in theirs."
"A bird doesn't mess up its own nest."
"You are all leaves of one branch and the fruits of one tree."
"If you don't want to be my friend, I'll bash your head in."
"Guests, like fish, begin to smell on the third day."

Questions regarding the Third Model Dimension (Relationship to "We")

1. Which of your parents was more open to contacts?
2. Which parent most enjoyed having company?
3. How were you drawn into your parents' social contacts? For instance, did they believe "Children should be seen and not heard"?
4. Were you a showpiece when your parents had company? ("Behave yourself when company comes"; "show them you're not stupid.")
5. What were the reasons for having (or avoiding) company? (Business reasons; obligations to relatives; company without making any real selections; a limitation on the number of guests because they cause disorder, cost money, et cetera.)
6. What were your parents' attitudes toward foreigners and members of different religious sects or political groups?
7. Were your parents socially or politically involved?
8. Did your parents belong to clubs, interest groups, citizens' coalitions, or labor unions?
9. What kind of people did your family prefer?
10. What is the significance of your career as far as relationships with other people are concerned?
11. Are you a bookworm, or do you prefer to be with other people?
12. Are you socially and politically active?
13. What people, organizations, and groups can you turn to when you have problems?
14. If you were separated or divorced, to whom would you turn? Where do you find comfort and security?
15. Which experiences come to mind when you hear these questions? What ideas do you associate with the relationship to "we"?

RELATIONSHIP TO THE PRIMAL WE (PARENTS—RELIGION/PHILOSOPHY OF LIFE)

BELIEVE IN GOD AND TIE YOUR CAMEL SECURELY

The faithful came in throngs to hear the words of the prophet Muhammed. One man listened especially attentively and devoutly, prayed with faith and fervor, and finally left the prophet when evening came. He was hardly outside when he came running back in and cried out with an excited voice, "O my lord! This morning I rode my camel to hear you, the prophet of God. Now the camel is gone. Far and wide, there's not a camel in sight. I was obedient to you, heeded your every word, and trusted in God's power. Now, O lord, my camel is gone. Is that divine justice? Is that the reward for my faith? Is that the thanks for my prayers?" Muhammed listened to these desperate words and answered with a kindly smile, "Believe in God and tie your camel securely."

Despite its uniqueness, the family does not create its own laws. The family is connected to the rules, orders, and laws set forth by social, religious, and political groups and institutions. In a closed society where there is only one generally recognized world order, the family and the individual adopt clearly prescribed tasks. The existing order determines the relationship to parents, siblings, contacts outside the family, opportunities for selecting a spouse, and the definition of friend or foe. Here the interpersonal relationships still follow relatively fixed laws, as, for example, in the case of the obligatory rules of hospitality among rural and nomadic groups in the Middle East. This custom follows closely the concepts set forth in the Koran, where it is said that guests are a gift from God. The value systems that determine the rules for interpersonal relationships and define one's connections with the environment are summarized as philosophies and religions. They not only comprise the socially regulative laws, but also determine a person's worth, the meaning of his life, and the goals he should strive to achieve. This dimension of human development is the relationship to the ideological construct that we term the "Primal We." This concept refers to the fact that our perceptions and actions all take place within a system that is culturally transmitted. Philosophical determinations influence not only our philosophical and religious activities, but also every scientific endeavor that the individual undertakes.

Religious interpretations have a special positional value. In contrast to other philosophies, they can be traced back to a seer or prophet. They correspond to a typical human need, a need for meaning (Frankl), a need for an overview in order to reduce insecurity (Secord and Backmann, 1964). As a result of these needs, people in all eras have been drawn to the founders of various religions. Even people who regard themselves as antireligious have been known to turn to "substitute religions."

The life of the individual and the organization of the family and other groups are influenced by concept systems of this type. The saying "Till death do us part," for example, is related to the Christian ethic and is supposed to protect the church-sanctioned marriage and the family stemming from it. But, most of all, education is influenced by the philosophical-religious image of man. Should a child learn to be obedient and serve his parents, as is called for in the Mosaic religions? Contemporary middle-class society, on the other hand, espouses a liberal view and encourages the child to be self-reliant, self-assertive, and independent. Here we should also mention the achievement-oriented education, as it is set forth in religion in the Calvinist doctrine and socially in the "climber mentality" of the self-made man. In their own attitudes to the "Primal We," the parents establish a model for their children. They shape religious fixations, the rigid adherence to religious dogmas, the kind of indifference some people like to display, the manifest repudiation of these themes, as well as an ambivalent relationship to religion and philosophy.

The person's relationship to the "Primal We" depends first of all on the parents' attitudes toward religion and philosophy. Since the parents take on almost godlike functions—at least in the child's first years of life—as being almighty, all-known, and invincible, it frequently happens that one's early experience of father and mother is carried over into one's expectations of God, or the "Unknown and Unrecognizable." Hence an unjust father or a repressive mother can lay the foundation for the idea of an unjust God or an unjust world or can cause the future to be perceived as obstructed, meaningless, or hopeless.

In contrast to the closed society I have just described, contemporary society is an open one. That is, various philosophical, ideological, and relious systems are no longer limited to definite geographic places, but exist simultaneously and in competition with each other. Today we can no longer look at the psychosocial norms valid in our group and consider them as absolute. Rather, we must compare them with other possible attitudes about values. In so doing, we do not lose our perspective; on the contrary, our perspective is broadened by the inclusion of other views.

PROGRESSIVE REVELATION

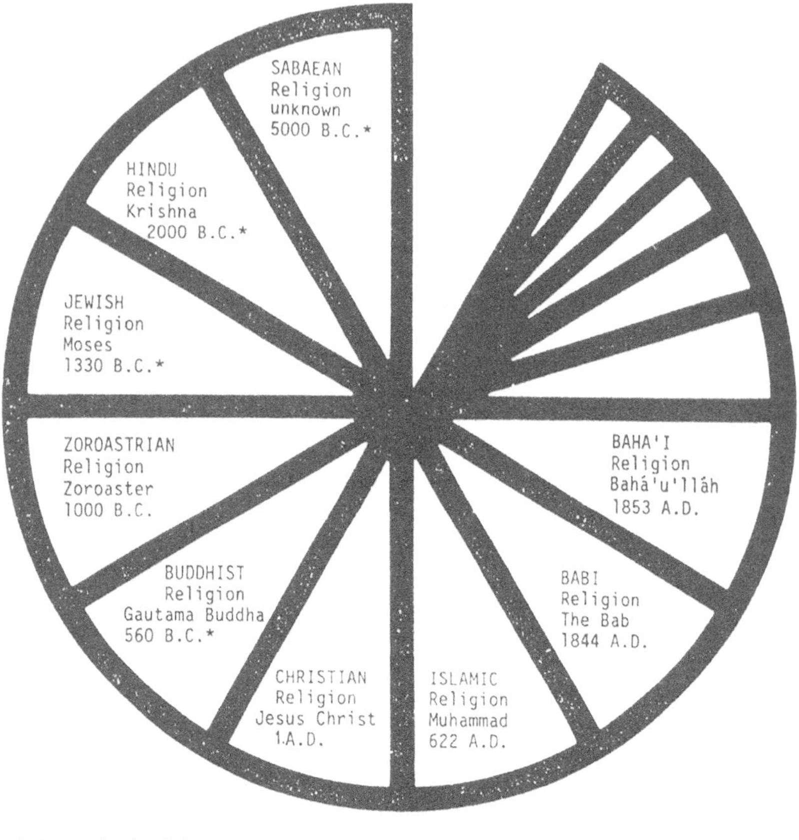

* Approximate dates.
Authorities differ on dates.

Concepts

"I have a positive attitude toward the world, can accept myself and other people, and trust that the crises that emerge from day to day can be solved somehow and give meaning to my life."

"I have to be suspicious of everyone and hide my talents under a bushel; I don't trust other people along the way; I question the meaning of my life."

Here, with primal trust and primal distrust, we may have come full circle after starting with the relationship to "I."

Questions regarding the Fourth Model Dimension (Relationship to the "Primal We")

1. Which parent put more emphasis on religious and philosophical questions?
2. Which religious and philosophical concepts did your parents represent?
3. Did your parents agree on religious and philosophical questions?
4. Did your parents have trouble with the rest of the world because of their religious and philosophical concepts?
5. Which parent prayed? Which one prayed with you?
6. Which parent was concerned about life after death, the meaning of life, the essence of God, et cetera? What did these questions mean to you?
7. What were your parents' goals in life? What is your goal?
8. How do religious and philosophical concepts influence you as far as child rearing, choice of spouse, and relationships to other people are concerned?
9. What were your childhood experiences with religious and political-philosophical events?
10. Do you consider yourself an optimist or pessimist?
11. Are you interested in religious, political, or scientific problems? Do you belong to a religious group or political party?
12. How do you get along with members of other faiths and representatives of other philosophic persuasions?
13. Are you preoccupied with death and life after death?

4. The Four Forms of the Model Dimensions in Positive Family Therapy

Man should know his own self, and know those things that lead to loftiness or to baseness, to shame or to honor, to wealth or to poverty

Bahá 'u' lláh

Just like the four areas of dealing with conflict, the four model dimensions can be applied to partner and family therapy. Using the various evaluations as a starting point, we can examine the areas in which each family member's personal experiences and interests have their greatest emphasis.

All of us stand within a tension field of relationships and connections. It is a field that is circumscribed by the four media for the ability to love. But, depending on our own experiences, these media are perceived differently by each of us. The individualist who is preoccupied with his own affairs and a concrete "You" and would like to dispense with a personal "You" or "We" nevertheless has a characteristic relationship to these areas, a relationship that is characterized, for example, by distrust. A thief who takes other people's possessions is, from this point of view, not basically disturbed in this relationship. Rather, he displays traits that lead him to the conduct that is contrary to societal rules. He can very well have an emphatic relationship to "I," as well as to a certain "You," a selected "We," and even to the "Primal We." Left out of the relationehip is the "You" of the victim or the societal "We" that disapproves of the theft and pronounces punishment.

Thus one medium of the ability to love, even a form of the relationship, can become a rival to the others; one can neglect one's partner because of preoccupation with oneself, neglect other people because of attention to one's family, neglect one's family and self because of other obligations and involvement in social issues, overlook actual needs because of strong emphasis on the "Primal We," or, under the demands of these needs, disregard the "Primal We." Emphasis on certain relationships can thus take on a symptomatic character, since disorders can develop from them because of corresponding external influences.

A married couple came for family therapy because of marital problems. The husband repeated in stereotypical fashion that he and his wife just weren't suited for each other and that the marriage was a real burden for him. His wife admitted that there were problems, but she was not ready to arrive at the same conclusion. She remained opposed to the idea of divorce. I inquired about the four model dimensions and got these results:

Relationship to "I"

Husband	Wife
The parents had had enough time for him, but were not always patient. To get their attention, he had had to excel at school and in sports. There were no siblings.	Because of their work, her parents had had little time for her. In her first years, she was taken care of by a nursemaid. It is important for her that her husband has a lot of time for her. She is the oldest of three children.

Relationship to "You"

His parents divorced when he was twelve. Prior to that, the father had had many affairs. Even the mother had consoled herself with a number of acquaintances.	Parents were together her whole life—in work, at meals, in bed. Rarely did the parents show physical affection in front of her, but she still considered theirs an ideal marraige.

Relationship to "We"

Both parents were very sociable. When there was a party, the child had been allowed to participate. Today he still likes to be with people. His job as a representative of his company is thus the right kind of work for him.	Parents had had few social contacts—business contacts with customers and social contacts with close relatives. When there were family gatherings, the child had had to keep quiet. In school, she had had only one good friend. Now she feels quite lonesome.

Relationship to "Primal We"

Parents were Protestant liberals. He had been confirmed.	Parents were conservative. As Catholics, they had gone to

Nonetheless, religion was treated mostly as a matter of form. For him, church was secondary. He regarded himself as an optimist; the most important thing for him was his career.

church every Sunday. She often wants to go to church, but her husband doesn't take her seriously in this matter. She is pessimistic, mainly because she feels very lonely

	Father	Mother
Time	+	+
Patience	–	+
Model	+ +	+

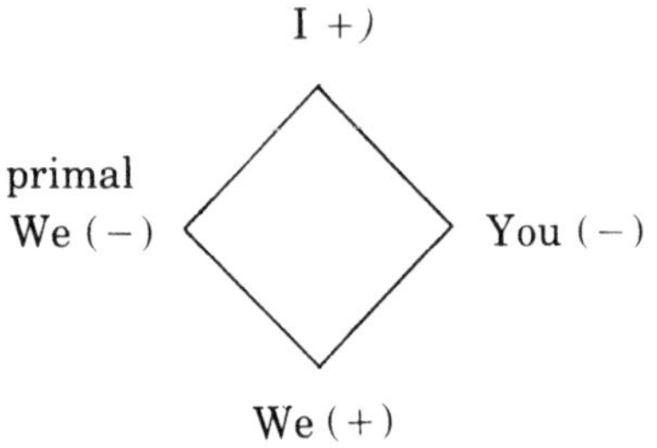

	Father	Mother
Time	– –	–
Patience	–	+
Model	+	+

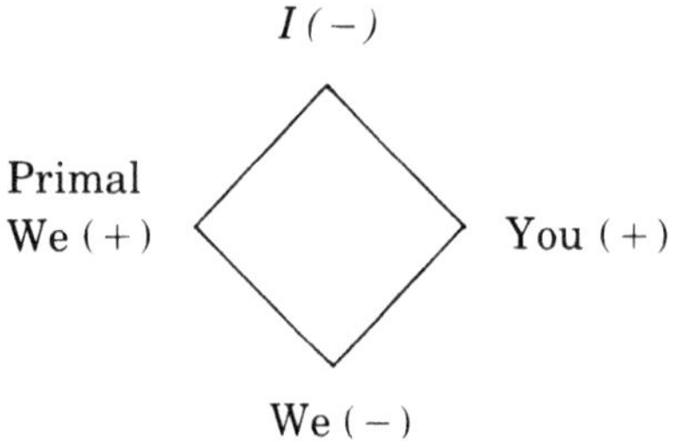

The four areas of the ability to love and the four corresponding model dimensions are thus especially important for Positive Family Therapy because they give an overview of the relational patterns that motivate a person within his group. They also provide an overview of the biographical conditions that extend back to the individual's family origins.

By means of the model dimensions, concepts are set forth in family therapy that have often not been expressed in this form before. Their expression often means that a member of the family is now ready to start therapy.

The model throws light on a person's social relationships. It describes the quality of his contacts. The concept "lack of contact" points to the fact that a certain type of contact, usually the relationship to

"You" and "We," is somewhat limited. Thus social norms (actual capabilities) can be switched on to filter one's social relationships; one dispenses with inviting people over, because they disrupt the normal routine and cost money. Company thus impinges on one's concept of frugality. Similarly, the relationship to "I" can be blocked by failure (industry/achievement) due to lack of support from the area of the primary capabilities. The relationship to "You" can be disturbed by conflicts dealing with sexuality, loyalty, and trust, just as unfulfilled expectations regarding honesty, justice, and hope can be placed in connection with one's relationship to the "Primal We."

In psychoanalysis, ego strength and ego maturity are central concepts. They are viewed as the criteria for the position of psychoanalytical indication and as the goal of the treatment. The concept of ego strength becomes problematic when strength is determined solely by the ego, while the other functions of social competence (relationships to "You" and "We" and the relationship to fantasy and the future) are disregarded. Naturally, it must be assumed that originally these social and prospective ego functions were also considered. But it seems typical that they do not appear explicitly. In this sense, the concept of ego strength adheres to the liberal will model of bourgeois society, whereby social relationships and the activity of fantasy are overshadowed by the achievements associated with conquering and controlling reality. There is ample evidence to assume that this is one reason why, until very recently, psychoanalysis dealt primarily with the individual and was concerned with strengthening the ego functions while the relational qualities in the family and social environment remained outside the picture: Why should one be concerned with these factors when psychotherapy had succeeded in strengthening the patient's ego? The social consequences of this method of procedure and the displacement of interpersonal symptoms were ignored. Treatment was directed toward a Nibelungen-like fidelity to the individual patient.

This also means that in family therapy the transference must be introduced differently than was possible in psychoanalysis. Through its emphasis on self-help, the focal and thematic orientation of Positive Family Therapy tries to avoid the transference neuroses in the relationship between therapist and patient. Transference takes place in many ways within the patient's social environment, an environment to which—during the time of the treatment—the therapist himself also belongs. For the therapist, it is a matter of registering the various transference relationships and investigating them in terms of the concepts involved.

5. Actual Capabilities

THE RIGHT PRICE

When King Anoschirwan traveled through the land with his people, he came to a desolate area in the mountains where there weren't even any pathetic little shepherd huts. The king's cook lamented, "Noble sultan! I am here to please your palate. But in our canteen we don't even have the littlest grain of salt. And without salt the food tastes terrible. Noble sultan, what should I do?" Anoschirwan replied, "Go back to the nearest town. There you'll find a merchant who has salt to sell. But be careful to pay the right price and not a bit more than is usual." "Noble sultan," answered the cook, "in your chest you have more money than anyone else in the world. What difference would it make to you if I pay a bit more for salt? That little bit won't amount to much." The king looked at him seriously and answered, "It is precisely the little things that grow into the injustices of the world. Little things are like drops of water that eventually fill an entire lake. The great injustices of the world began as little things. So go and buy the salt at the usual price."

ACTUAL CAPABILITIES FROM THE TRANSCULTURAL POINT OF VIEW

The goal of this segment is to specify the capabilities and conflict susceptibilities of people in a concrete way, and to determine the rules that direct our day to day actions. When we have problems with ourselves, our spouse, and our environment, when we don't know what to do, and when we react to conflicts in mental and psychosomatic ways, we must investigate the nature of the conflicts. I may have been motivated in part by the fact that to a certain degree I live in a transcultural situation. As a Persian (Iranian) I have lived in Europe since 1954. This perspective made me aware of the importance of psychosocial norms in socialization and the development of spiritual and interpersonal conflicts. With American and Europeans patients, as well as ones from the Middle East, I found that behind the symptoms there were usually conflicts that went back to a series of recurring behavioral norms. I tried to collect these norms, assemble them into concepts that relate to each other, and to set up an inventory for describing the central areas of conflict. I called these behavioral norms *actual capabilities*. I established this term because it includes norms that operate in our everyday interpersonal relationships and thus have a continuing and timely significance. Differentiation analysis starts with the actual capabilities as potentials for both development and conflict. We do not deal with some mysterious concepts known only to the specialist, but with norms and concepts that everyone encounters every day. What is really behind it all when we get angry, feel furious with someone, retreat with great indignation, feel wronged, or want to jump out of our skins: I have delved into this question and have tried to grasp the conditions behind the problems and conflicts of my patients and clients. Step by step, over a period of eight years, I set up the actual capabilities in their present form. At first I was struck by the psychotherapeutic significance of politeness and honesty. These two categories offered a guideline for completing the inventory of actual capabilities. This inventory was repeatedly checked and enlarged through what I discovered in the course of my practice.

THE COURSE OF A DAY

6 :15: Get up quietly so my wife isn't disturbed. Have shut off the alarm fifteen minutes early so it wouldn't go off; then into the shower; say good morning to my youngest son, who is already awake. Rinse out the bathtub and the glass we use for brushing our teeth; make sure there's no hair in the comb [actual capabilities in operation: promptness, politeness, cleanliness].

7:15: Leave the house without having seen anyone except my youngest son. I tell Wolfgang to keep quiet so that the rest of the family can keep on sleeping; close the door quietly.

9:00: I go back home to have breakfast with my wife and Wolfgang. I talk to him about school and exchange a word with my wife now and then. In the morning, things usually go their merry way without any big disputes [contact, politeness, punctuality, achievement].

9:30: I go back to the office.

12:30: Back home for lunch. It's usually not ready yet, and this aggravates me, because I like to be able to rest for an hour after lunch if I can [achievement, punctuality, time, patience].

1:00: Lunch with my wife, Wolfgang, and Christopher. Minimal conversation at the table. This time I'd like to have a more personal conversation with Christopher than I ususally do and thus don't talk about school if I can avoid it. Because I was mad last night that they'd left all the lights on and the windows wide open with the furnace running, I tell them all about it. My wife has nothing to say about it except "Your father is a real Scrooge." But electricity costs money, and so does oil for the furnace. I don't see why they keep all the lights on even when no one's at home. I think my wife is very unfair to me [*contact, achievement, politeness, frugality, justice*].

1:30–2:00: A short nap in my room, during which time my wife takes all the phone calls. She gets paid by my company for doing this [*time, achievement, frugality*].

2:00: Back to work [*promptness, achievement*].

5:30: After work I go to my health club to swim 1,000 meters so I can stick to my fitness program [*achievement, in relation to one's body*].

6:45: Come home. The food isn't on the table yet. I've bought some food on the way home and ask my wife to fix it [*promptness, patience, time, trust, contact*].

7:00: Supper with my wife and Wolfgang. We all help clear the table. Wolfgang is gotten ready for bed. When he's in bed I pray with him and say goodnight [*contact, politeness, order, religion/faith*].

8:00: Watch the news on TV. My wife sits there with the dog, who is very sensitive to noise and jumps and howls if he hears bells or sees the weather map. This used to upset me, but today I just keep quiet. Sometimes my wife grabs hold of the dog and takes him out of the room before he starts his "act." Most of the time I sit alone in front of the TV. My wife putters around somewhere or watches TV on the set upstairs. Without my knowing it, she had bought it for our son, even though she knows we don't have money for things like that [*contact, patienct, politeness, achievement, frugality*].

9:00: Dead tired. Start to doze off in front of the TV, so get ready for bed. If I see my wife I say goodnight and then turn in [*time, contact, politeness*].

During the day I hardly see my two older children, and I rarely see them at night either, because they have their own friends and don't feel comfortable in our tense family situation [*achievement, contact, doubt*].

Journal of a Forty-eight–Year–Old Patient

If we start with the interpersonal relationships, then look at the standards for evaluating ourselves and others, examine the criteria for upbringing and psychotherapy, and finally clarify the conditions that lead to the known psychic and psychosomatic disorders, we see that behind these disorders—to a certain extent as deep structures—there is a lack of differentiation about the behavioral patterns of ourselves and other people. In depicting psychic and psychosomatic disorders, we use concepts like excessive demand, overwork, or stresses. But when we say there are stresses behind the disorders, we have not yet said what kind of stresses they are. Usually one tends to attribute them simply to work, but actually there is a whole spectrum of ideas and behavioral patterns that have become potential conflicts, i.e., are predestined to cause psychic and psychosomatic disorders. These attitudinal and behavioral patterns can be described by using an inventory of psychosocial norms that are likewise effective as developmental dimensions and conflict potentials.

We can name the following behavioral attributes: punctuality, cleanliness, order, obedience, politeness, honesty, loyalty, justice, industry/achievement, thrift, dependability, exactness, conscientiousness, love, patience, sexuality, trust, confidence, hope, faith, doubt, certainty, and unity. We label these behavioral attributes as actual capabilities because they are rooted in the human being as capabilities and are actually effective in day-to-day life.

The day's events that are outlined above provide an example of how important the actual capabilities are. Everyone can examine his day in terms of the actual capabilities involved. In the preceding example, one can recognize a number of psychosocial norms that reflect important qualities in the family and allow us to determine the father's position. This focus on the actual capabilities shows that certain themes are repeated in typical fashion (achievement, punctuality, thrift, contact, patience); they are played out in the family situation, of course, but the members of the family don't really give much thought to them.

The actual capabilities can be divided into two categories, which we call *secondary* and *primary capabilities*.

SECONDARY CAPABILITIES

The secondary capabilities are an expression of one's ability to recognize, to be aware. In them are reflected the achievement norms of the social group to which one belongs. They include punctuality, cleanliness, order, obedience, politeness, honesty, loyalty, justice, industry/achievement, thrift, reliability, exactness, and conscientiousness.

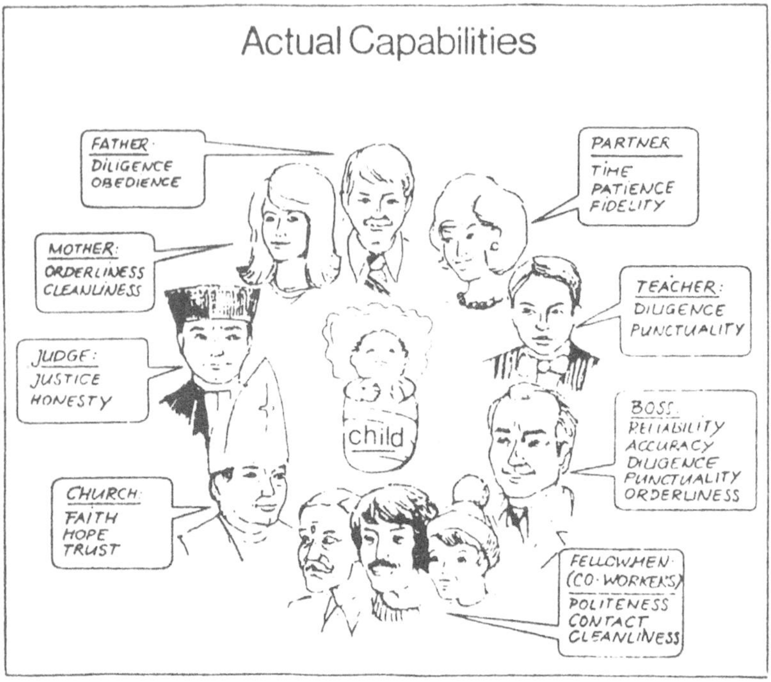

In day-to-day descriptions, evaluations, and mutual judgments, the secondary capabilities play a decisive role. When a person finds another person nice or likable, he frequently justifies his opinion this way: "He's decent and orderly, the kind of guy you can depend on." On the other hand, a negative assessment usually goes like this: "I dislike him because he is sloppy, late for appointments, unfair, rude, and stingy and doesn't show much ambition." It is equally common that experiences can influence one's mood and physical well-being. Pedantry, disorder, ritualized cleanliness, lack of hygiene, excessive demands for punctuality, tardiness, compulsive conscientiousness, or irresponsibility, for example, can lead to psychic and psychosomatc problems as well as to social conflicts: "Whenever I think of my boss reproaching me for mistakes I didn't make, I start to tremble and feel ill. Later I get a headache and upset stomach," says a twenty-eight–year–old employee with psychosomatic disorders. The actual capabilities involved are justice and politeness.

THE PRIMARY CAPABILITIES

The extensive affective resonance of the secondary capabilities can only be understood on the basis of emotional relationships. The primary capabilities deal with the ability to love. This capability, too, develops out of interpersonal relationships, whereby the relationships to significant persons, particularly to the father and mother, play a central role. The primary capabilities comprise categories such as love (emotionality), model, patience, time, contact, sexuality, trust, confidence, hope, faith, doubt, certainty, and unity.

In terms of content, the primary capabilities are oriented according to experiences that were made in view of the secondary capabilities. On the basis of the primary capabilities, the secondary capabilities find their emotional resonance: "I can't trust my husband now that I've found out he has had an affair" (actual capabilties: trust and loyalty).

We conceive of the primary capabilities as the prerequisites for emotional ties, yet if we do not understand them as individual capabilties, but as integrated parts of closer interpersonal relationships, we find that they form a typical chain of developments that follow this sequence: unknown capabilities, anxiety, aggression, imitation, faith, doubt, hope, trust, confidence, patience, certainty, love, and unity.

The members of the family pass through this developmental chain, but usually they don't occupy the same position at the same time. In one person, faith, doubt, and hope can correspond to the unknown capabilities in another person. One person's doubt can correspond to another's certainty. One person's position in the developmental chain can prevent some conflicts, but it can also cause conflicts when two people are going through different phases. For instance, one person might react aggressively and skeptically to a partner's disorder or one person's anxieties might provoke such a sense of hopelessness in the other person that these conflictual limitations destroy their love.

Each of the actual capabilities can be put into operation in an active or a passive way. Active means to be punctual/tardy, to be orderly/disorderly, to be honest/dishonest, et cetera. By passive we mean here: "How do I react to the other person's

demands for punctuality or tardiness? How do I deal with my family's disorder or its wish for order? Can I put up with my partner's demands for justice or with their injustice?

The position of the family member does not just depend on which actual capabilities are expressed, but on whether it actively demands or passively expects them. Frequently the recognition of this double-sidedness is the decisive event in solving the conflict. One doesn't just speak out on behalf of justice, but when necessary, is also able to put up with injustice without being destroyed by it.

6. Microtraumas: The So-called Little Things

The highest form of wisdom is kindness.

—Talmud

As a result of microtraumatic experiences in one's upbringing, one is more sensitive and receptive to the details of those areas than to other ones. Just as a steady stream of droplets can eventually hollow out a stone, so the day-to-day experiences with the actual capabilities create areas of reduced resistance. Hence for one person, tardiness can unleash a lot of unrest, anxiety, and aggression, while another person can be upset by his or her mate's rudeness, messiness, demands for punctuality, or lack of reliability. If different attitudinal and behavioral patterns confront each other in a relationship, there can develop conflicts that accumulate as microtraumas, which in turn form neuralgic points in the structure of the personality. Against this background, a continuing emotional stress can set in, which then leads to psychic and psychosomatic disorders, inhibiting communication within the family. For example: "If I don't clean up my room, it always means 'I don't love you anymore.' That thought always put me into a panic. Today I am terribly pedantic, and this often gets me into trouble with my husband and children," says a thirty-nine–year–old housewife with inhibitions, social anxieties, difficulties in dealing with people, and marital problems. In the first instance, the actual capabilities involved are order, trust, and contact: in the second case, obedience and politeness are the main themes.

These contents reflect relational aspects of the partnership or the group. The husband's desire for order is more than just his personal notion of what orderliness should look like. Along with other actual capabilities, his need for order describes a rule that is characteristic for his marital and familial relationships. In other words, we find that the relationships are crystalized in the contents of the actual capabilities.

The actual capabilities can be realized in an unlimited number of different attitudes, values, experiences, and behavioral patterns. The concepts (for example, "Orderliness is half of life"; "If you save something, you have something"; "What will people say?"; et cetera), however, are the contextual, situational, group-specified or personality-linked characterizations of these actual capabilities. When we look at them more closely, we can determine that concepts frequently do not just refer to individual actual capabilities, but comprise various actual capabilities in varying degrees of importance.

Actual capabilities do not just appear in the terms we set up, but also in the form of synonyms, concepts, and paraphrases. Hence, instead of using the word *order*, we say, "Don't mess up my things. Clean up your room. Don't leave anything lying around. Hodgepodge! What a mess! A pigpen inside and out."

What's important is that we discover the actual capabilities operating behind the day-to-day events and behind what the partner says and does. This is particularly important in family therapy, in that the critical behavior must first be identified before the family rules can be redefined, using the critical behavior as the starting point. This requires that we realize that the individual capabilities can take on all sorts of diguises.

Hence there isn't just one form of disorder. It expresses itself in many ways: As rational, factual order: "Everything must be cleaned up so we can always find what we're looking for." As traditional order: "Everything must be in its place, just as we've always had it." As intuitive, imaginative order: "There is only one place for this vase—the niche in front of the winter garden." As romantic order: "I can't live in a constricted atmosphere. My surroundings must convey a certain warmth, and I can't sense that in a sterile place." As outer order: "When company comes, the house must be tidy." As inner order: "I could care less how I look. What matters is that I feel at peace with myself."

Even the messiest of people have their own order and personal sense of order. We must learn to recognize it.

Definite reflections of actual capabilities are hidden in the most seemingly unimportant behavioral patterns: the mother who is contantly fussing with her son (cleanliness); the father who often looks at his watch (punctuality); the grandmother who tries to control the kids by giving them dirty looks (politeness/obedience); the daughter who is scolded for butting into her parents' conversations (openness, politeness, obedience).

7. Making Contents Concrete

It is better to have a friend in the marketplace than gold in the coffer.

—Leone Da Modena

We don't limit ourselves to general observations like "authoritarian family home," "strong parental ties," or "rigid or relaxed upbringing," and we do not just speak of "conflicts of self-esteem," "inferiority complexes," "sexually disturbed," "suffering from burnout," "improperly raised," "hooked on religion," "incapable of change," "living under a lot of stress," "hole in the ego," "deficient in contacts," "phobias," or "a far-reaching but vague superego." Rather, we attribute concrete contents (actual capabilities) to inner psychic events and one's interactions with other people.

As an example, in the case of depression we don't just investigate the depressive symptoms or a priori established key conflicts; intead, we look for behavioral areas where the corresponding conflicts are involved. In the case of anxiety, we don't concentrate on the theme of anxiety per se, but on the series of conditions that work to trigger the anxiety. A patient, for instance, always developed anxieties when she had to wait for her husband in the evening. In terms of content, her anxiety was focused on the psychosocial norm of punctuality. Isn't the next step then to deal with this area?

In corresponding cases, where the depressive symptoms also stood in the foreground, "mourning training," "justice training," "contact training," "politeness training," "honesty training," et cetera were carried out in an analogous way. Here—along with the meaning that Positive Family Therapy has in and of itself—there developed the possibility for intergration with other psychotherapeutic directions. From the view of psychoanalysis, one could summon associations with punctuality and then work out these associations. In this connection, the conversation could deal with the problem of separation and the infantile separation anxieties. This content orientation seems particularly meaningful for short-term therapy that focuses on a particular theme.

For behavioral therapy, the precise examination of the contents of the anxiety—fear in a punctuality situation—would be an important aid for establishing an appropriate hierachy of anxieties, which we could then designate as a "punctuality hierarchy" (Peseschkian, 1977).

Various psychotherapeutic approaches can thus make good use of the tools of Positive Family Therapy without losing their own standing as independent approaches.

8. The Significance of the Actual Capabilities

If everyone sweeps in front of his door, the whole City will be clean.

The secondary and primary capabilities (actual capabilities) are not simply labels or passing occurrences. They appear as engrained and actual rules, roles, and attitudes about interpersonal relationships and as more or less adequate behavioral directives for the individual. They are marked as specifically human capabilities in the course of socialization, are acquired, internalized and, to some degree, effectively employed. Examples are "My son's dirty hands spoil my appetite" (twenty-six–year–old mother with a nervous stomach) and "When I find out my daughter has gotten a bad grade at school, I get pains around my heart and break out in a cold sweat" (thirty-four–year–old mother of two).

While industriousness is an important trait for one person, another person might place more importance on order, punctuality, politeness, honesty, thrift, justice, exactness, et cetera.

In the personal and collective areas, we are confronted by the effects of the actual capabilities every day—namely, when a marriage takes place or is dissolved, when a friendship disintegrates, when someone is fired from his job, when the relationship of groups or people with each other becomes the origin of a conflict.

The actual capabilities become specific traits of a group by means of the influence of tradition. Among other things, tradition can exert considerable influence on the relationships between the in-group and the out-group (cf. Peseschkian, 1970, 1971, 1977).

Particularly in the case of vegetative-functional disorders and neuroses and psychoses associated with behavioral disorders, one finds that the psychotherapeutic and medical literature abounds with references to the individual actual capabilities. Freud (1942) cites sexuality and cleanliness. Jung (1940), Kuenkel (1962), and Frankl (1959) emphasize the importance of faith. Fromm (1971) speaks of hope. Mitscherlich (1967) arrives at the importance of the demands for achievement and motivation. Dreikurs (1970) points to the connection of success, prestige and exactness with learning problems. Bach and Deutsch (1962) point to the importance of an open relationship (honesty) in the partnership. Erikson (1966, 1971) formultates a sequence of virtues that are built up according to the individual developmental stages of the individual and the maturity of the psychic functions. He lists trust, hope, will, determination, loyalty in one's adolescence, and concern and wisdom in one's adult years. But the systematic connection between these components is not given much consideration (cf. Peseschkian, 1977, pp. 94–102).

Discoveries show that displacement in the area of the secondary and primary capabilities leads to a limitation of one's sense of value. That means that the individual overemphasizes a capability that he is adhering to at the moment. He is so blinded by its value that he is oblivious to other values and capabilities: "The only kind of person who counts with me is one who behaves well. I don't care how successful he is; if he is not well mannered, I just can't look up to him," says a fifty-three–year–old woman with headaches and circulatory problems.

The disorders that are represented by the actual capabilities can develop from a dissonance within the secondary capabilities themselves (one can be industrious but not orderly), within the primary capabilities (one can trust other people but not himself), or in the connection between primary and secondary capabilities (one can be orderly but not patient).

From this point of view, vegetatively functional disorders, neuroses, and psychoses can be interpreted as a reaction to conflict between primary and secondary capabilities and thus as the result of insufficient differentiation.

9. Actual Capabilities as Signs of Transcultural Differences

Every new answer raises a new question.
—Oriental wisdom

The list of actual capabilities in their current form developed step by step over a span of ten years. At first, I had been struck by the psychotherapeutic importance of politeness and honesty. After I had become sensitive to these two psychosocial norms, I was able to see again and again in my own behavior, in the things I experienced in my family, and in my dealings with other people and patients norms that were very important psychosocially. Then there were areas that, as virtues, were the goal of upbringing and developmental dimensions on the one hand, but on the other hand were often found in connection with disorders, aggravations, complaints, problems, and illnesses.

The categories of the primary and secondary capabilities offer a guide for completing the inventory of actual capabilities. The inventory was checked again and again through my observations in clinical practice and was examined for supplementary possibilities and with the goal of determining whether the actual capabilities can be used as an aid in describing the conflicts under observation.

As we all know, we tend to make friends with people who think the way we do, who have the same ideas about things as we do, and whose tastes and interests do not differ significantly from ours. If our group is formed in this way, there soon develops a fixed repertoire of answers and, consequently, a common base of things that are obvious to everyone in the group. After a while, a person hardly has anything new to say and is satisfied to keep hearing and repeating the same things just out of habit and complacency. But if people of different cultures and types of upbringing get together, tensions can easily develop. They stem from the fact that various behavioral patterns and expectations come into conflict with each other. Keep in mind, after all, that one member of a group soon learns to be polite. He then tries to avoid being aggressive with his associates and, at the same time, tries to be tolerant of the occasional rudeness of other members in the group. Another person, however, can find that this is a false and deceptive attitude, since he learned early on to come out and say what is on his mind. The interaction between these two people alone is enough to cause conflicts that can even destroy the harmony in the entire group.

In Western society, we see a tendency to emphasize the secondary capabilities, such as the achievement principle. At times this means that the primary capabilities, like contact, are neglected. In the Midde East, however, emphasis tends to be placed on the primary capabilities—that is, the capabilities that center on contact. As a result, various secondary capabilities are obviously neglected.

As an example of transcultural differences, let's take a look at how we deal with the actual capabilities of time, punctuality, and patience. Every person has the ability to determine how he divides up his time. But the opinions we hold about these divisions of time depend in great part on our particular cultural point of reference. A highly organized industrial society is based on the punctuality of its members, but in a peasant society people can divide up their time in less rigid ways. They can place more value on patience than on punctuality. This stems from their particular situation. They have to learn to wait and adjust to the rhythms of nature. Thus various systems require different attitudes toward time. None of these divisions of time is necessarily better than the other ones. Each has its points of conflict: emphasis on punctuality in connection with the stress symptoms of industrial society; generously structured time divisions in connection with the fatalism of population groups in the Middle East. The relationship to industry/achievement corresponds to this difference: between affluence, production, and a consumer society, on the one hand, and a self-sufficient, less production-oriented way of life on the other.

It is equally tense when different relational systems come up against each other. Aid for developing countries, industrialization, and—in the opposite direction—flight from the cities, folklore, and alternative life-styles are all examples of the confrontation between various life-styles.

Individual life-styles and the class of various concepts produce typical conflicts—often because extreme forms of a primary or secondary orientation—fail to pay attention to the totality of a person's capabilities. The ability to achieve (ability to recognize; secondary capabilities) and the ability to be emotional (ability to love; primary capabilities) do not exclude each other, but complement each other. We can thus conceive of a utopia with social conditions where a person can develop all his capabilities into a harmonious relationship. The person is thus able to achieve, but without losing touch with his feelings and his need for interpersonal relationships. At the same time, he can develop deep emotionality and an ability for close contacts without sacrificing the development of his productive capabilities.

Not everyone must be as orderly as a bookkeeper, as punctual as a stonemason, as exact as a tailor or as clean as a surgeon. Set free from the situation and time context that gives them their full justification, the capabilities become a caricature and, even more, a conflict potential. A surgeon scrubs several times before an operation, each time for anywhere from three to five minutes. If he follows the same ritual at home and demands it of his family, this practice, which is appropriate and even necessary in the one situation becomes a farce. It has no function; the child will rebel against the rule, the wife will become aggravated, and family life will be upset.

10. Using the Differentiation Analytical Inventory (DAI)

It is better to know nothing than to learn nothing.
—Oriental wisdom

The actual capabilities can be determined by means of the differentiation analytical inventory. The DAI thereby becomes an inventory of concepts that are relevant to individual, familial, and culturally determined conflicts.

The DAI can be carried out in the therapeutic situation and also by individual family members within the framework of self-help. We thus get as many differentiation analytical inventories as there are members in the family. In these inventories, self-assessment always goes under the "I" column and one's evaluation of his partners and their behavior are placed in the "other partner" columns. Diagnostically, one can combine these various evaluations of oneself and others into a differentiated conflict diagram. Even family members who are absent—deceased parents, a divorced spouse, a family member who refuses to take part in the therapy sessions—can be indirectly included in the dynamics of the concepts held by the family and the individual. We call this process Virtual Family Therapy.

The assertions in the DAI are not absolute judgments. Rather, they are subjective evaluations, relative in regard to specific partners. The individual standards of the family members are compared with each other.

PROCEDURES FOR USING THE DAI

Data: Twenty-three–year–old secretary, married for five months. Symptoms: functional disorder of heartbeat, sinus arrhythm, paroxysmal tachycardia, stomach trouble, phobias, and depression.

The patient said she was troubled by things in her marriage and

Differentiation Analytical Inventory (DAI) Short Form

Actual Capabilities	Patient + –	Partner + –	Spontaneous Answer
Punctutality			
Cleanliness			
Orderliness			
Obedience			
Politeness			
Honesty Sincerity			
Fidelity			
Justice			
Diligence Achievement			
Thrift Economy			
Reliability Exactness			
Love			
Patience			
Time			
Trust Hope			
Contact			
Sexuality Sex			
Belief Faith			

complained, "Although we understand each other in a physical sense, we aren't suited for each other. We're such different people." We than carried out the DAI.

The questions read: "Are there conflicts in the area of punctuality (order et cetera)? Which of you puts more value on punctuality (order et cetera)?" Depending on the particular case, modifications of the questions are possible.

The behavioral areas are marked in such a way that + + + designates the highest subjective evaluation of a category and – – – the lowest evaluation; + – means indifference towards the behavioral area to be assessed; + +, +, and – –, – are further levels of the subjective evaluation. The second column represents the patient's self-evaluation of the actual capabilities. The third column is the patient's assessment of the partner; as needed, additional columns can be included for other important people. The last column is reserved for comments.

Differentiation Analytical Inventory of a Twenty-three–year–old Patient

Actual Capability	*I*	*Partner*	*Comments*
Punctuality	+ + +	+ −	When I pick up my husband, I can easily wait a half-hour for him. But if I happen to be late, he becomes impatient.
Cleanliness	+ +	+ +	No problems. Neither my husband nor I is a slob.
Orderliness	+	+ + +	In my opinion, a house should look like it's lived in. My husband thinks it should look like a picture in a catalogue.
Politeness	+ + +	+ + +	We both think it's important to be considerate of each other. I don't want to hurt my husband, and I have never yet heard an insulting word from him.
Obedience	+ −	+ −	I think people should adjust to each other and make some sacrifices. But when someone like my father demands absolute obedience, I don't like it at all. My husband feels the same way. He still refers to his father as the "general."
Honesty	+ −	+ +	My husband is more likely to say what he thinks. But that is hard for me sometimes, because I don't like to hurt someone's feelings.
Faithfulness	+ +	+ +	There are no problems here. I think fidelity is very important to both of us.

Justice	+ + +	+ + +	I think I'd get very upset if my husband treated me unfairly. He is as sensitive on this point as I am.
Thrift	+ −	+ +	On the basis of my earnings, I treat myself to what I need.
Industry/ Achievement	+ + +	+ + +	I think we both want to be successful in our careers.
Dependability/ Reliability	+ +	− +	As far as his job is concerned, my husband is dependability personified. And, when it concerns him, he puts a premium on dependability. But when I expect some dependability from him, it just doesn't work.
Patience	− −	+ −	This is something I don't always have.
Time	+ + +	− − −	We don't have much of a family life. My husband works the night shift. When I leave in the morning, he's asleep, and when I get home, he's not there.
Trust/Hope	−	+ +	When I think about our marital problems, I tend to view it as all black. I hope we can change things in therapy.
Contact	+ + +	−	My husband is a loner. He has inhibitions that others wouldn't be able to accept. We live pretty isolated, although I like to be with people. I suffer quite a bit because of this.
Sex - sexuality	+ + +	+ + +	I like it, and I think my husband does, too.

Faith/ Religion	+ −	+ −	We're both Protestant but have never given much thought to this issue.

Punctuality, orderliness, politeness, time, and contact were shown in the preceding case to be conflict potentials and areas of constant emotional stress.

Punctuality

The husband's laxness in this area—an area of great importance to the patient—is felt to be an injustice. His tardiness is viewed as a crisis in their trust.

Order

Here we found two different concepts of order. The patient feels she's hemmed in by her husband's pedantic nature. For the patient, the conflict that arises here is directly connected to the possibility of feeling comfortable in their shared space.

Politeness

For both partners, politeness has a stabilizing function. The ritualistic courtesy prevents them from bringing their conflicts out into the open. Politeness thus becomes a sign of blocked aggression and causes the conflict to be turned inward.

Time

Here we see that social and economic factors are involved ("If my husband didn't have to work the night shift . . .). The time the husband can spend with his wife is subjectively perceived by her as a kind of allowance.

Contact

Here, too, there are diverging concepts. The patient interprets her husband's lack of contact as a way of protecting himself (imagined differences in status between the two). She herself appears to be quite strong in this area and develops desires that cannot be fulfilled in the interplay with her husband's concepts.

A potential for conflict in this area could be traced back to the life history of the patient and her husband (basic conflict). Here the DAI was again used, with the question "What did your parents put most value on? Who placed more importance on punctuality (orderliness et cetera)?" On the basis of this analysis of the actual and basic conflicts, we were able to grasp the conflict situation.

As a form of Positive Family Therapy, the therapy was conducted as partner therapy and was terminated after fifteen sessions that spanned six months. When the treatment ended and when there were a follow-up examination a year later, the patient proved ot be free of symptoms. She commented that the quality of their marriage had clearly improved: "The turning point for me was when I got away from the idea that we weren't suited for each other and when I discovered the day-to-day problems that were at the root of our tensions."

11. Actual Conflict and Basic Conflict

"While my mother stooped over to get every little piece of fuzz, my wife lets the dust lie till its a half-inch thick."

In order to understand a conflict, we must know how it developed and which inner and outer conditions created the susceptibility for this development. We look into the life history of the individual family member and the relationships that stamped the image of their personalities. In so doing, we eventually discuss the concepts that already existed before the patient's birth—concepts that to some extent shaped the social form in which he grew up with his particular capabilities. In terms of their temporal and conditional sequence, we can distinguish between two conflict areas: the actual conflict and the basic conflict.

ACTUAL CONFLICT

This term refers to conflict situations produced by actual problems, like excessive demands in one's work, marital problems, difficulties between children and parents, et cetera. These conflict situations also can trigger an existing acute symptom. With respect to content, the actual conflict expresses itself primarily through the behavioral categories of the actual capabilities, the four areas for dealing with conflict, and the four model dimensions. These contents, grounded in the subjective value system, lead to conflicts as soon as their consequences go beyond the limits of what the individual can tolerate:

> *A child comes home from school and tosses his books into the corner of the front hall. The mother has seen this from the kitchen and becomes terribly angry. She would like to summon the child to pick the books up, but her aggravation is so great that she is speechless. She begins to tremble and then bursts into tears. Her anger is based on her notion that orderliness is extremely important. This idea is based on what we call the basic conflict.*

BASIC CONFLICT

The actual conflict doesn't come by chance, as if out of the blue. It develops very slowly and finally reaches a threshold where the susceptibility of the family or one of its members becomes a mental or physical disorder. It is much like the drop of water that causes the barrel to overflow. We do not just investigate that one drop that triggered the actual conflict, but also the many drops that filled the barrel in the first place. This means that we trace the person's development back to his early childhood and to the developmental condictions in the family—back over several generations, if possible. The equipment for this journey into the past is again the tools of Positive Family Therapy.

By getting at the basic conflict, we come to understand the conflict susceptibilities in the personality structure as well as in the family structure. It is primarily the theories of psychoanalysis and depth psychology that deal with the basic conflict. The goal of the therapy is to become aware of the conflict and to work through it.

According to Positive Family Therapy, the central elements in the basic conflict are concepts that are closely linked to the personality and the family game rules. These concepts also represent a predisposition toward the conflict. Since the concepts are acquired early in the individual's development, we call them basic concepts. In the life of the individual they are a theme that reoccurs in many variations. This is why Positive Family Therapy does not seek to restructure the entire personality, but only the concepts, and then primarily the basic concepts. In so doing, we do not just focus on the therapeutic process in the individual alone. Rather, we see it as a process that takes place in both the individual and in his relationships to groups around him.

Why did the mother in the preceding example think that throwing things in the corner was so terrible? Why did she get so angry about it? We must look for the answer to this question in what the mother learned in the past. The following scenarios are plausible: the mother was scolded and punished for being messy when she was a child, other people were responsible for keeping things in order when she was little, and she thinks that should still be the case, or she was given a lot of attention for her orderliness then, so continues to give it a lot of importance now.

An analysis of the family situation shows that the mother imitates her own mother's behavior (tradition) and unconsciously identifies with her. The emotional involvement is based in part on the fact that the parent made sacrifices for her husband, the child, and the household and neglected her own interests and needs (relationship to "I"). As a result, she regards the child's behavior as a sign of ingratitude and injustice. She focuses her attention on the child partly because her husband has little time for his family ("You") and because the mother hardly has any contact with other people ("We"). The mother's hopes are thus directed toward the child. She clings to assumed ideas of orderliness and obedience—ideas that are deeply rooted in her as the conditions for being a "decent person" ("Primal We").

Positive Family Therapy does not just look at how people were and how they now are. It also tries to envision what they can become and how these possibilities can be realized.

Notions that seem unchangeable and unalterably linked to the personality can be made relative to terms of the individual's life story. The process includes becoming aware of the ideas, filling in gaps in the person's memory, and reexperiencing his developmental history. But the process includes more than this: By looking at the conflict-laden ideas and behaviors in terms of their background conditions, the family members can gain a greater degree of control over them. They learn that they can influence the conflict. The goal is to understand the behavioral areas (actual conflict) as biographically conditioned (basic conflict) and alterable (relationship to the future).

12. The Three Stages of Interaction

THE HAKIM KNOWS EVERYTHING

A man lay bedridden with a serious illness, and it appeared that his death was near. In her fear, his wife summoned a hakim, the town doctor. The hakim tapped around on the patient and listened for more than a half-hour, checked his pluse, put his head on the man's chest, turned him onto his stomach and then his side and back, raised the man's legs and torso, opened his eyes, looked in his mouth, and then said with a great deal of conviction, "My dear woman, unfortunately I must give you the sad news that your husband has been dead for two days." At this very moment, the ailing man raised his head in shock and whimpered anxiously, "No, my dearest, I'm still alive." The wife gave her husband a hefty slap on the head with her fist and replied angrily, "Be quiet! The hakim, a doctor, is an expert. He ought to know."

—Persian story

In his personal development as well as in his marital and family relationships, the individual goes through three stages: connectedness, differentiation (discrimination) and detachment.

THE STAGE OF CONNECTEDNESS (ATTACHMENT)

This is based on the unborn child's dependence on his mother. It is loosened by a social symbiosis after the child's birth. The child is now dependent on the care and attention he gets from his social environment. He demands patience, time, and attention and requires physical and social contact. For their part, the parents feel tied to the child through love, hope and responsibility. But the need for connectedness is something man feels his entire life. This accounts in large part for his search for a marriage partner, his desire to be with other people, and the cohesiveness of the group, as represented by the family.

If the need for connectedness becomes the dominant behavior in the person—a type of behavior extending over long periods of time and occurring again and again in his interpersonal relationships—we refer to it as a *naive-primary* behavior. This type of reaction springs mainly from an overprotective upbringing in which the primary capabilities occupied the forefront. The naive-primary type corresponds to the depressive structure of neuroses. The chief reaction is the escape into loneliness or the escape into contact, which offers solidarity and shelter.

Concepts

"I can't do it alone."
"The others have to help me."
"If I don't get some help, it's a lost cause."

THE STAGE OF DIFFERENTIATION

Differentiation is a basic principle of both physical and mental development. In socialization, the stage of differentiation is marked by the acquisition of socially desired behavior. This happens in the differentiation of the person's ability to recognize and learn and in the formation of the secondary capabilities, which enable him to control nature and to assert himself socially. At the same time, there is differentiation in one's ability to love. That is, we learn how and to whom we can reveal our feelings and in what social forms we can satisfy our urges. In other words, through differentiation our feelings take on a social shape. This process comes about through the confrontation with the structures that we find in our environment. In the stage of connectedness, general concepts like optimism, pessimism, self-acceptance and self-repudiation take on their shape. In the differentiation stage, however, the specialized concepts and behavioral norms develop: "Wash your hands"; "Get up"; "Behave yourself"; "Learn something"; "Save your money"; et cetera. This take place through direct instructions, by example, and by rewarding desired behaviors and ignoring or punishing undesired ones. As a form of adaptation to the environment, differentiation can help a person have a life that is free of friction. But it can lead to problems if the individual structure of differentiation does not agree with the other differentiation structures. A further complication can be expected if the socially desired role behavior does not make allowances for existing urges. If the differentiation gains the upper hand in an imablanced way, we speak of the *secondary reaction type*. Located in the area of this secondary type—which is oriented to the secondary capabilities—we find the compulsive neuroses structure. The compulsive person uses his "superdifferentiation" to ward off threatening urges and to force them into the tight corset of a pedantic life-style. Matter-of-fact relationships are given more attention than real emotional participation. The secondary type is characterized by an escape into activity.

Concepts

"I can handle everything alone."
"I don't need help from anyone."
"Let other people work for you"

THE STAGE OF DETACHMENT

Within the development of the individual, a specific unity can be achieved at each developmental level. *Unity* refers to the integration of the capabilities into an individual personality. Associated with it is an autonomy that takes on more and more importance until the individual reaches maturity. At the early stages of his development, a person is quite dependent in terms of connectedness, and even later on he needs to be guided by certain rules. But as he grows older, he needs this outside information ot a lesser degree. He has adopted this information as concepts and makes his decisions with them in mind. At the same time, this means he can detach himself from other people, can find for himself the information he needs, and can then take on responsibility for himself. Here we are referring to a stage of detachment that characterizes the maturing and mature personality.

Detachment does not just mean that one turns away from an object or a person. The succession of detachment and connectedness makes it possible to establish contact with other persons and groups; that is, one can widen his field of values and try new decisions, but perhaps also reevaluate old values. Many people swing back and forth between detachment and connectedness. They want to be independent but find they can't deal with their independence. Or they want the love and attention of a marriage partner but at the same time tend to evade it because of their desire for freedom. We refer to this kind of person as the *double-bind type*. In general terms, the double-bind type of behavior corresponds to the hysterical neuroses structure. People affected by it are influenced by sudden forces and new possibilities outside themselves and appear to be unpredictable with themselves and their environment.

Concepts

"I can do it all alone; but someone must help me."
"I want to, but I don't want to."
"I don't like it when you help me, but I'm not happy when you don't help me either."

The developmental conditions for the basic conflict were presented here in terms of their typological aspects. Types are essentially abstract summaries of common traits. But, in reality, things are a lot more colorful. There are fewer pure forms. Instead, we find a lot of mixed forms in various degrees and shades. One of the major differences between the typical attitudes and behavioral patterns on the one hand and the common typologies on the other is that we understand the reaction type dynamically on the basis of the conditions surrounding its origin. Constitution and predisposition play a secondary role. That is, the particular form of upbringing, the typological categorization, is not determined by fate, but can change over the course of time.

QUESTIONS REGARDING THE THREE STAGES OF INTERACTION

To determine the stage of interaction at which a partner is at a particular time, the following questions are posed. For the stage of connectedness: "Does my partner (at this particular time) have a need to be with me?" "Does he need my love and attention?" "Has he developed an intense emotional relationship with me?" For the stage of differentiation: "Does my partner lack information?" "Does he need my advice?" "Does he need my opinion in order to arrive at a decision?" The stage of detachment represents the diminishment, change, or disintegration of emotional ties. We speak of disintegration when a partner tries to put forth his own ideas, when he wants to reach his own decision. We then ask, "Does my partner want to make a decision for himself, even without my help?"; "Does my advice limit his personal freedom?"; and "Is he demanding independence for himself?"

Each of these stages meets with a stage of expectation in the other person. One must ask himself, *Do I expect my partner to stay with me, help me, feel emotionally tied to me, and show his gratitude?* (Connectedness); *Do I need to give my partner advice, to influence his de-*

cisions, or to warn him about things? (Differentiation); *Do I expect independence from my partner? Would I prefer not to be responsible for him? Do I feel it is right to leave him to himself?* (Disintegration).

Example of a Situational Analysis Based on the Three Interaction Stages of Connectedness, Differentiation, and Detachment.

Connectedness	Differentiation	Detachment
The twenty-eight–year–old working wife looks forward all day to spending time with her husband in the evening.	When the husband comes home, he complains, "I see that the kitchen is a mess and the kids' things are lying around all over the place. At times I wonder why people get married."	The husband sits down in front of the TV. The wife retreats to the bedroom.

THE STAGES OF INTERACTION IN POSITIVE FAMILY THERAPY

The stages of interaction play a role in the relationship between the therapist and the patient's family as well as in partner and family relationships. During the connectedness phase, the therapist is like a host for the patient's family. He accepts them as they are. It is helpful for him at this point to remember that the members of the family, just like he himself, have a lot of capabilities in common. He identifies with the family and its members, but without getting sucked into the maelstrom of the conflicts. He learns to understand why the family feels compelled to seek refuge from the symptoms and why the symptoms are so important to the people involved. By using the tools of Positive Family Therapy, the therapist structures the information given to him by the family.

The connectedness is related to the conflict theme, which is identified through the tools of Positive Family Therapy. For a certain period of time, this theme becomes a focus for mutual identification and the family's attempt to regain earlier connections to their own past within the family (regression). Individual problem groups like psychosomatic, depressed, and schizophrenic patients who normally do not seem receptive to therapy provide information through their verbal and nonverbal behavior; this information, in turn, is useful to the therapist.

This is particularly the case in the family therapy situation where the entire family is present and provides insight into their relationships. But it also holds true for the direct therapist-patient relationship. To cite an example: A twenty-five–year–old patient, who had been diagnosed as schizophrenic, complained right at the beginning of the first therapy session because the light was on in the conference room. He scolded me for this, and this remark proved to be the beginning of our mutual connectedness. At first it revolved around the subject of thrift, and as a result, we were, as psychiatrists would say, able to converse with "good affective rapport."

At the stage of differentiation, the therapist presents these realizations as information, interpretations, and prescriptions. By means of his "translations" and counterconcepts, areas of common agreements and clear delineations are drawn between the interests of the family members, i.e., the family subsystems. The members of the family can "try on" new concepts offered to them and identify with them on an experimental basis. They can test game rules that provide suitable solutions and alternatives.

At the detachment stage, there is an increasing distance between the patient's family and the therapist. The latter becomes more and more an observer of the process taking place and intervenes in a regulatory way only when it seems necessary. In the differentiation phase, the therapist was the one who provided initiative, alternative suggestions, information, and structural assistance. But now these activities have been taken up by the patient and his family. To an ever increasing extent, they take on the tasks associated with self-help.

THE THREE INTERACTION STAGES FROM A TRANSCULTURAL PERSPECTIVE

These three interaction stages can be observed in every interpersonal relationship. Certain patterns can be viewed as cultural characteristics. An example of this is the Mideast connectedness, a relationship that is so deeply rooted that parents send their children thousands of miles away to school and still know that, despite the distance, the children are still dependent on them and the clan. There is a kind of social umbilical cord that is almost untouched by the distance. Gifts, personal signs of attention from home, financial help, visits, a constant exchange of letters, and frequent phone calls help maintain the family connections. But in the Western industrialized societies, independence and autonomy are the desired qualities. There is a trend toward detachment. Connectedness is viewed as a sign of dependence, immaturity, and the inability to stand on one's own feet and adjust to seemingly necessary separations. Until around puberty, connectedness is emphasized. But after that there is often an abrupt detachment, with the parents' saying, "You're old enough. You must know what you're doing now." It's usually more common, however, that the adolescent initiates the detachment: "I'm old enough and can stand on my own two feet." Clinging too closely to one's family is regarded as a threat to one's independence.

With regard to the naive-primary, secondary, and double-bind types, this approach was mainly thought of as a structural aid for the therapist. But in the three interaction stages it is resolved into relationship problems that people can actively deal with. This change from a diagnostic to a therapeutic point of view is a chief characteristic of Positive Family Therapy. It is given its due in both the contextual process as well as in the five-phase treatment strategy outlined in "Part VI: The Five Steps in Positive Family Therapy."

Part VI.

The Five Steps in Positive Family Therapy and How They Operate

THE MAGICIAN

The mullah, a preacher, wanted to get some nuts for his wife, because she had promised to cook him fesenjan, a dish prepared with nuts. In the joy of anticipating his favorite dish, the mullah reached deep into the nut jar and grabbed as many nuts as he could reach with one hand. When he tried to pull his arm out of the jar, it was stuck. As hard as the mullah pulled and twisted, the jar would not release his arm. He cried, groaned, and cursed as a mullah really shouldn't. But nothing helped. Even when his wife took the jar and pulled on it with all her weight, nothing happened. His hand remained stuck in the neck of the jar. After many futile attempts, they called their neighbors for help. Everyone followed with great interest this play that was going on in front of them. One of the neighbors took a look at the problem and asked the mullah how this accident had happened. With a pathetic voice and moans of desperation, the mullah told of the mishap. His neighbor said, "I will help you if you do exactly as I say."

"I promise to do everything you say, if you can just free me from this terrible jar."

"Then shove your arm farther into the jar."

This seemed strange to the mullah, for why should he put his arm farther into the jar when he wanted to get it out ofthere? But he did sas he was told.

The neighbor continued. "Now open your hand, and drop the nuts you are holding." This request upset the mullah. After all, he wanted the nuts for his favorite dish, and now he was supposed to just drop them. Reluctantly, he followed his helper's directions. The man now said, "Make your hand very small, and pull it slowly out of the jar."

The mullah dropped the nut, and, behold, without any trouble, he pulled his hand out of the jar. But he wasn't completely satisfied. "My hand is free now, but where are the nuts?" At that the neighbor took the jar, tipped it over, and let as many nuts roll out as the mullah needed. Wide-eyed and with open mouth, the mullah watched and said, "Are you a magician?"

—Persian story

The core of Positive Family Therapy is the five-step process. I'd like to illustrate the logic of this process with an example taken from everyday life: When we get upset over the rudeness, injustice, or dishonesty of our mate, we tend to feel bad inside, to complain openly about him, to discuss him and his weaknesses with other people, or to simply withdraw. We will no longer see him as a person with a manifold capabilities, but simply as the rude one, the unjust one, or the liar who has hurt our feelings with his poor behavior. We are neither willing nor able to consider the person's fine qualities, which we would have otherwise found positive and pleasant. Our unhappy experiences with him lie like a shadow over our relationship with him. The relationship has thus taken a destructive course that adheres to very typical game rules: We are prepared only to look at him as the "bad guy." Every dealing with him deteriorates into a power struggle, an emotional scene, or resignation. Communication is blocked. Things finally get so bad that in order to punish him, we actually limit our own goals and withdraw. We retreat into a corner and solidify the disturbed situation. This change of events can lead to psychic and psychosomatic disorders. It represents a typical way of dealing with conflict. Corresponding to it are the five stages of psychotherapy, which we present as a model for the therapeutic process:

1. stage of observation/distancing;
2. stage of inventory;
3. stage of situative encouragement;
4. stage of verbalization;
5. stage of goal expansion.

The five stages are oriented according to the four ways of dealing with conflict, and their goal is an expansion of the repertoire of possibilities for dealing with conflict.

For each of these stages in the treatment there are a number of stories, concepts, and parables at our disposal. They can be applied to the particular needs of the treatment. Within the five-phased Positive

Family Therapy, they are an aid for the patient's methods of dealing with fantasies. At the same time, they help the therapist develop connections to fantasy and intuition.

Each of the five steps speaks to the person as a social being and draws him into the human community in which he developed and in which his conflicts originated. They stimulate his ability to help himself. In other words, Positive Family Therapy goes back to the family group in which the patient lives. If the family group is not readily available, the therapy draws on people who replace that family in some way or other. The therapeutic process then runs its course on two levels:

LEVEL ONE

At this level, all intervention is carried out by the professional therapist. His professional competence is a prerequisite, but the therapy can vary in content, depending on the partner's individual and professional socialization. The following four factors characterize psychotherapeutic competence in terms of Positive Family Therapy:

a) *Sympathetic understanding:* In psychoanalysis, this is known by terms like empathy, transfer/countertransfer (Beckmann, D., 1974, 1978). Control over this happens by means of the therapist's own self-discovery. He appears here as the "patient" and is confronted by the reality and conditions of his own concepts.

b) *The ability to use the tools of Positive Psychotherapy:* This means to be able to think in terms of their contents, concepts, and models of Positive Psychotherapy and to apply them in a flexible way, always oriented toward the particular needs of the patient.

c) *The application of other psycho and social therapeutic processes in which the therapist has been trained:* Here a wide range of possibilities can be used—elements from psychoanalytic procedure (Freud) and behavior modification techniques (Wolpe, 1962; Innerhofer, 1978), methods of conversational therapy (Rogers, 1962; Tausch, 1974), individual psychology (Adler, 1947), Gestalt therapy (Perls, 1951), transaction analysis (Berne, 1964; Harris, 1975). et cetera.

d) *Ecological thought:* This extends from individul psychotherapy to community psychology. Family therapy stands at the central point.

For the therapist, the five-phased model is a guideline that helps him structure the therapy. It is a platform from which he can observe the course of the treatment. It is an orientation aid by which he can make adjustments in his own therapeutic approach. It enables him to move in the alien world of the patient and the patient's family without getting lost in it himself.

LEVEL 2

Here activities are carried out by the designated patient and his family group. This is the level of self-help. Here the patient gives up his role as patient. He begins to redefine his relationships within his group, his family. At this level, the resulting changes are played out, such as the shifting of individual and interpersonal symptoms, the appearance of a newly designated "patient," and the working out of particular answers. The therapeutic competence that was required at the first level is the goal of the therapy at the second level. The patient learns to use the tools of Positive Family Therapy, thinks about the previously used processes in his lay therapy and the concepts underlying them, gains conscious access to his family and social ties, and increases his ability to understand in an intuitive, sensitive way. He thus acquires the skills that he needs to conquer his conflicts. For the patient, the five stages are a way to help him get an overview of the therapeutic process and to actively take over activities of self-help within their sequential order.

There is constant interplay and exchange between the two levels. Through this exchange one should come to learn that changes in the family and redefinitions of roles can lead to new concepts for dealing with old conflicts and disorders.

1. The Stage of Observation/Distancing

THE PHARISEE AND THE PUBLICAN

Jesus told this parable to some who trusted in themselves that they were righteous and despised others:

Two men went up into the temple to pray, one a Pharisee and the other a tax collector. The Pharisee stood and prayed thus to himself: "God, I thank thee that I am not like other men, extortionists, the unjust, adulterers, or even like this tax collector. I fast twice a week, I give tithes of all that I get." But the tax collector, standing far off, would not even lift up his eyes to heaven, but beat his breast, saying "God, be merciful to me, a sinner!" I tell you, this man went down to his house justified rather than the other; for everyone who exalts himself will be humbled, but he who humbles himself will be exalted.

Luke 18: 9–14

As persons involved in the conflict, the members of the patient family have, as a rule, lost their distance from the conflict. This is true for neurotic, psychosomatic, and psychotic disorders. The people involved in the conflict act much like someone who is standing so close to a picture that he almost touches it with his nose. He sees only a small segment of it but he sees this segment very clearly. Yet he doesn't see its subject or color context. He has lost sight of the picture as a whole and has thus also lost its meaning.

This example illustrates the cognitive function of the observation/distancing stage. To illustrate its social and emotional meaning, I can cite another example: On a cold night, two hedgehogs had a problem. When they got too close to each other to get warmed up, they poked each other with their needles. But if they got too far away from each other, they froze. It was crucial that they be close enough to warm each other,but also far enough away so as not to poke each other.

THERAPEUTIC FOCUS

The therapist establishes ties with the patient and in some cases also with his family (connectedness). He takes time for them, invites them in for discussions, observes the situation that the session poses for him, and listens to what they have to say. During this time, he structures this information and questions the feelings he has developed in regard to what the people have presented to him. Here, too, behavioral analysis (Schulte, 1974; Kanfer and Saslow, 1965, interaction analysis (Bales, 1950; Innerhofer, 1974), and the analysis of psychoanalytic transference are helpful. Who takes the *initiative* within the family? How do the other family members respond to it? Do they obstruct the initiatives or do they go along with them? We don't acquire information simply from what the patients say, but also from their nonverbal behavior (cf. Innerhofer, 1978): *Pauses* (absence of visible reactions, obstruction of an initative, not wanting to know more, waiting for reaction); eye behavior (eye contact, orientation of the eyes, breaking off eye contact, looking at the floor, et cetera); *motor movements* (getting up, turning away, et cetera); and *expression* (tone of voice, mimicry, pantomining, attitude). How does the therapist himself perceive the form of interaction? We thus try to exhaust all available sources from which we can get situational and anamnetic information about the symptoms and their accompanying behavior. With observation, something very important happens within the therapeutic situation: Each member of the family is able to present himself without fear of a negative reaction or even punishment by the therapist.

Parallel to this, the therapist tries—initially for himself—to develop a general *positive reinterpretation* of the disorder. It should include the significance the illness has for the patient and his family. This process helps the therapist distance himself from his own structures of perception and his own models of thought. At the same time, it avoids repeating the neurotic concepts of the patient. The therapist conveys his thought experiment to the patient and his family, within the framework of an appropriate situation. He passes on an interpretation that best facilitates the most effective change of perspective. The success of this process, however, should not falsely lead one to impatiently remove the positive reinterpretation from its connections to reality; it can, after all, be experienced in some cases as a kind of cynical scorn. (If problems emerge here, the therapist can use the four model dimensions to reflect on this own problems.)

By providing alternative concepts, the positive process leads to new points of departure that can change the family's game rules fundamentally. With this change, something else happens. The family learns to deal with its conflicts in new ways and to give up its pathological fixations. This is the first step toward self-help. The patient's family is given instruction about the five stages of Positive Family Therapy and thus get an overview of what they can expect from the therapy. A framework for the therapy is set up, which can in given cases also include time limits:

Depression

Example: A thirty-four–year–old patient had sought psychotherapeutic treatment because of severe depressions. For long periods in the initial discussion he described—often repeating himself to the point of exhaustion—his feelings of inadequacy and his mental depression. In so doing, he clarified the vicious circle that his thoughts and feelings moved in without having any alternatives. The therapist tried to present a positive interpreetation: The depression was an expression of his strong emotional involvement. It was thus a matter of finding out what the patient felt so intensely about. This gave the patient the opportunity to stop describing his feelings and to concentrate on depicting the situation that tormented him so. For some time now he had had both a wife and a girl friend and now stood at the crossroads, having to make a choice, since his "game" had been discovered. His attempt to solve the conflict consisted of his negating it: "If only I hadn't gotten married!" or "If only I hadn't met my girl friend!" He made use of the tactic of sticking one's head in the sand in the hope that the danger would thereby go away by itself. To this the therapist gave a sensitive, positive reinterpretation: "I think I can understand how much you are suffering from all this. You say the situation causes you pain. But can't it also be fortunate when someone has two women like you do?"

This question astonished the patient. As he said later on, he had expected to be reprimanded for his "immoral" action. Not only his preconscious wish for punishment, but also the self-punishment that was contained in his depressive symptoms were thwarted by the positive reinterpretation. He now recalled many a night in the past years of his marriage when, rejected by his wife, he had longed for the warmth and tenderness of another woman. He also remembered the lusty fantasies of his puberty—fantasies of being pampered by two women at the same time. The initial conversation thus took on a new dimension: out of the previously "unproductive" patient there developed a "productive" patient who was able to establish connections to his contradictory feelings, fantasies, and experiences and to relinquish them in front of the therapist.

INSIGHT INTO PSYCHOSOMATIC CONNECTIONS

For many people, it is hard to recognize the background of the symptoms, particularly when they themselves or close relatives or friends are affected by them. It is thus a question of getting from the symptom to the conflict. A patient has every right to expect that the doctor will explain to him how the findings originated. In the same way, I try to explain to the patient and his family just how his symptoms developed out of conflicts. I have found that this kind of instruction, which can occur quite early in the treatment, has a positive effect on the motivation in the patient's family. To do this, I often us the story of a made-up conflict that contains elements of the origin of the psychosomatic illness:

Imagine a likable, successful young man. He has a charming, conscientious, and tidy wife. But he also has a nice, pretty girl friend he likes to be with. The man feels twofold happiness. The wife is happy, for she knows nothing about the girl friend. The girl friend is happy, because she thinks the man prefers her to his wife. Everyone is happy. But their happiness stands on shaky ground. Let's imagine the case a bit further on. After a while, the girlfriend demands, "Either her or me. I need a clear decision from you." The wife becomes suspicious, finds out about his tricks, and also demands, "Her or me." The man is right in the middle; rather, he's at the fork in the road. He feels tugged at by both women, yet is afraid of the consequences. What is this man experiencing? One can easily imagine that he tends to be upset and is easily excited, aggressive, or reclusive; he doesn't want to hear anything about anything and develops depression. Suddenly he gets headaches and perhaps wakes up from nightmares and can't get back to sleep. At the office, he can become nervous and unable to concentrate. But it's also possible that this whole aggravation effects his stomach. As a result of the upset and all the conflict, heart trouble and even rheumatic and asthmatic problems can set in. The young man, who had sexually satisfied two women previously, has perhaps been abandoned by one of them by now. The world no doubt seems incomprehensible to him.

The main feature of the disorder in this example is that the man stands in conflict between two possibilities that each have their good and bad aspects. That doesn't have to happen only in the sexual realm. Conflicts can develop in all sorts of areas: in one's job; in relationships with one's parents, children, and colleagues; and in one's religion and philosophy.

Even examples from suggestion research can contribute to our understanding of the psychosomatic processes that arise from the connections between thoughts or expectations and physical responses. The information given to the patient's family is a therapeutic attempt to modify their concept of the illness and to help them see through to the meaning of the psychotherapeutic process.

SELF-HELP

The patient, and in some circumstances also his family, begin to develop the competence for self-help. For a period ranging from one to four weeks, the emphasis is once again on connectedness and positive reinterpretation. The following measures are aids in the process:

> *Observation:* Watch the behavior of your partner. Write down what upsets you and what makes you happy. Describe this situation carefully. Questions to guide you: With whom and when did you feel angry or depressed? What cheered you up and made you feel happy? What do you like about your partner? What don't you like? What brought you together, and what keeps you together? The generalized discomfort will be put into a shape that makes it possible to gain new points of view and to usher in a relearning process in terms of the family and its relationships.
>
> Writing it all down serves a function much like a valve: the patient deals with his conflict, but does not intensify the external conflict situation.
>
> *Refrain from Criticism.* While you observe your partner, don't criticize. Instead of criticism, observe your mate, who does not take enough time out for you, is fussy and rude, et cetera. Through objective observation and the avoidance of criticism, the conflict can be uncovered. Day-to-day interaction is now perceived from a new point of view. Familiar habits, such as the criticism game, are abandoned, at least for a while, and the attitudes and expectations linked with them are not fulfilled. For the family member who risks taking this step toward self-help, the stage of observation/distancing requires time. He must allow time for his partner, and he must have patience to accept his partner as he is.
>
> *Write Down the Course of the Day/the Course of the Week:*

Write down in detail how you spend your day. Do the same thing for last week. This is an exercise in self-control. One can discover imbalances as well as areas of interest and areas one has neglected. Frequently this exercise already uncovers the central concepts of a person and his group.

Practice Celibacy and Faithfulness: In the case of sexual disorders or stubborn marital conflicts, there is a three-week period when there should be no sex (cf. Masters and Johnson, 1964). A prerequisite for this is the verbal agreement of the marriage partner. This measure should create some distancing from the couple's sexual habits. Tenderness, on the other hand, gestures of love and attention that arouse pleasant feelings in the partner (touching, stroking, embracing, kissing, intimate conversations, et cetera), should be given more emphasis. To avoid adding to the marital problems and to avoid escape reactions and guilt feelings, the marriage partners agree that during the time of the therapy of self-help, there should be no extramarital relationships on either side.

Settle the Problem with the Partner: Problems are private matters. Don't discuss them with a third party. Instead of talking about anxieties, aggression, and depression, make notes about the conditions under which they occurred. Often something balloons into an insurmountable problem only when it is carried out in a large forum. It's better to limit the problem to those directly involved in it. Often a conflict never gets settled—not because the people involved wouldn't have been able to deal with it, but because other people can't forget it.

Note the Actual Value and the Target Value: Delineate your conflict by using the Actual Value and the Target Value. Open the way for behavioral alternatives. The relearning process is mostly hampered by the fact that the people involved only see the conflicts and nothing else. Their reactions to conflicts appear to be determined by fate. It is our goal at this point to help the patient discover alternative attitudes and behaviors for himself. The patient presents real conflict situations. The actual value reflects his reactions and contains the patient's concepts that are involved. The target value comprises the counterconcept that appears to the patient as a practicable alternative.

Cope with Distress: Many people are afraid of being confronted with their conflicts and problems. Because of them, these people feel unsure and upset; they suffer when they can't avoid these conflicts. But psychotherapy and family therapy demand precisely this kind of confrontation. It's much like going to a dentist who is drilling a bad tooth. This worsening of the pain can be avoided only to a limited degree. But then the doctor fills the cavity and the pains stop. A family that wants to start therapy finds itself in a similar situation. Its members are suffering.

But the intervention from the therapist does not promise an immediate release from the troubles. Actually there is a provisional worsening of the situation, an increase of distress. But this is not the result of an error in the therapy. It is an important step in the treatment and is the best evidence that a central neuralgic point has been touched.

2. The Stage of Taking Inventory

THE TWO HALVES OF LIFE

A Mullah, the proud owner of a boat, invited the village schoolmaster for an excursion on the Caspian Sea. The schoolmaster lolled about under the canopy and asked the mullah, "What kind of weather will we have today?" The mullah checked the direction of the wind, looked up at the sun, unwrinkled his brow, and answered, "If you ask me, we's going to have a storm." Horrified by this reply, the schoolmaster made a face and said cricitally, "Mullah, didn't you ever learn grammar? It's not we's, *it's* we're.' *" The mullah responded to this reprimand with nothing but a shrug of his shoulders. "What do I care about grammar?" he asked. The schoolmaster was at his wits' end. "You don't know grammar. That means half your life is down the drain." Just as the mullah had predicted, dark clouds developed on the horizon, a strong wind whipped the waves, and the boat bobbed around like a nutshell. The waves drenched the boat with mountains of water. Then the mullah asked the schoolmaster, "Have you ever learned to swim?" The schoolmaster answered, "No. Why should I learn to swim?" Grinning from ear to ear, the mullah replied, "Well, in that case your whole life is down the drain, because our boat is going to sink any minute now."*

The stage of inventory places its main emphasis on the differentiating process. At this point the therapy deals with more than just the areas linked to the undesired behavior. A number of capabilities now come to the fore so that the members of the family acquire new criteria for evaluating each other. Figuratively speaking, they come to realize that a peacock doesn't just have ugly, wrinkled, leathery feet, but also has marvelous feathers.

It is essential that the family group be able to separate out these qualities and to experience the biographical roots and relativity of their evaluations.

THERAPEUTIC FOCUS

The therapist uses the tools of Positive Family Therapy. He can do this in such a way that he shows the patients the models and explains and researches them systematically by using these models. The patients become facile at using the tools of Positive Family Therapy as a means of self-help. This process is particularly suited to patients who have trouble getting in touch with their feelings and talking about their conflicts. To a certain extent, they first now learn the language they need to express their problems. While these patients had assumedly learned in childhood how to express an endless number of factual details and to suppress their feelings, the tools of Positive Family Therapy now help them overcome these deficiencies. The tools offer them the possibility for developing an operative mode of thought and for establishing connections with the feelings and conflicts they have neglected.

Example: The stage of inventory in the thirty-four–year–old depressed patient mentioned previously yielded the following picture:

> *Areas for Dealing with Conflict:* The patient had strong desires to withdraw from areas that were conflict-laden (wife, girl friend). When he compared his wife and his girl friend, he tended to prefer the latter because of her physical attractiveness (body, means of the senses), her career independence (achievement), and her way of getting along with other people (contact).
>
> *The Four Model Dimensions:* There were strong ties to his mother. The patient had been an only child. The father was busy in his work, so the patient had taken over the role of being his mother's confidant. On the other hand, opportunities for contact with other people seemed to be limited. The patient was affiliated with the Catholic church.
>
> *Actual Capability:* At the beginning of his illness, the patient was fixated on the areas of industry/accomplishment, punctuality, and conscientiousness. Coinciding with his depression, he began to neglect these areas. In connection with his connection with his mother, he was ambivalent toward the religiously motivated relationship of fidelity. Already in the early days of his marriage, fidelity had been a problem. But at that time it was the conflict of fidelity to his wife as opposed to "fidelity" toward his mother. His wife kept the house clean and in good shape—she was even too finicky, he felt. His girl friend, on the other hand, had a career of her own (industry/achivement), earned more money than his wife, and was financially secure (frugality).
>
> *Actual Conflict and Basic Conflict:* There was a problem with

fidelity, combined with a compulsion to make a choice (fidelity—doubt). In many ways, the patient felt obligated to other interests (the situation and good reputation of his family; the generation task transmitted to him from his parents, to keep his family intact; the moral principles of his religion, which demanded unconditional fidelity; and the social demands for achievement, which, as sexual achievement, suggested he maintain contact with a "successful" girl friend).

Reaction Type and Interaction Analysis: Naive-primary form of reaction with elements of the double-bind type.

On the one hand, the patient was a successful man in terms of middle-class standards. In a certain respect, he was justified, indeed obligated, to also document his success in the area of his marriage (detachment). In looking for a girlfriend he chose a woman whose characteristics flattered him. On the other hand, he was obligated by his parents' commandment to at least give the outward impression of having an intact family. Furthermore, he was faced with the religious-moral obligations toward his wife and two children (connectedness).

Concepts

"If you can do something, you are something."

"If you have something, you are something." (criterior for comparing the two women.)

"Till death do us part" (religious concept in reference to fidelity).

"What will people say?" (concept of loyalty toward parents; internalized politeness; fear of reaching one's own decision, since it might not be accepted by other people).

GUIDELINES FOR SELF-HELP

Areas for Dealing with Conflict: Write down the areas in which your problems come to a head. How does your mate work through his problems?

The Four Model Dimensions: Who was your model? What kind of relationship did your parents have to you and to each other? What was their relationship to other people and groups? Where did they stand on questions of religion and world view? How do you see the four model dimensions for your partner?

Actual Capabilities: Go through the DAI for yourself and the partner involved in the conflict. Describe the corresponding situations as a way of elucidating your assessments.

Concepts: Which motto or concept seemed to determine things in your parents' house? What is your guiding principle today? What are your partner's concepts? Who is your favorite writer? Which of his writings occur to you right now, and what do they say to you? Who treated you before? How do you, your marriage partner, your parents, and the doctors treating you relate to psychotherapy?

Misunderstandings and Interaction Analysis: In which areas do you and your mate have disagreements that have contributed to your conflict? What stage are you at now (connectedness, differentiation, detachment)? What stage is your mate at?

3. The Stage of Situational Encouragement

IRON IS NOT ALWAYS HARD

While treating a patient who had expressed similar thoughts, I described the following image. It made her very pensive and caused her to reassess her relationship with her marriage partner. "Look at this piece of iron," I said as I showed her a cast iron sculpture on my desk. "This iron is gray, tough, cold, and sharp-edged. When it is heated, it loses these characteristics. It is no longer gray, tough, cold, and sharp-edged, but glowing white, fluid, hot, and without a definite form. To a certain extent it has taken on the qualities of the fire."

For the patient, this meant that her husband's "sharp-edged" manner was not an unchangeable personal trait, but depended on the situation and on the patient herself. Because of his profession, he had less time for his wife than she wanted. She reacted to this with complaints and open refusals. As a result, the man sought other partners from time to time, aggravated his wife with his excessive frugality, and more and more frequently avoided her. To put it into images: The iron had grown cold. In order to forge it again, it had to be reheated. This was a task that the woman had to take up within her therapy.

By dealing with things that we find positive and pleasant, it is easier for us to also keep sight of things we regard as unpleasant and negative. This is, to sum it up in a few words, the basic principle of situational encouragement in Positive Family Therapy. Many people tend to act in one typical, one-sided way. They accept desired behavior of their partners without comment and talk only about behavior they don't like. Behind this kind of reaction there is the notion that only a "pessimistic" view can give a true picture of reality. Going along with this, such people tend to view an optimistic attitude with scepticism, even if it is an optimistic view of the same event that they see pessimistically. They say optimism is mere self-deception and falsehood. Besides the tradition that this pessimistic concept has, it also serves an important function: IT IS A SHIELD AGAINST DISAPPOINTMENT AND FAILURE. Because they have forseen the demise, their logic seems to say, they are no longer vulnerable to it.

THERAPEUTIC FOCUS

Situational encouragement and the positive process accompanying it are of central importance in family therapy. I have observed again and again that when a family concentrates only on its problems, the situation gets so bad that it is no longer one that can be controlled. But if we focus on the things that hold the family together despite all the problems, we encourage the family members to recall the positive relationships that have long been forgotten. We thus create a common ground where we can deal with the family conflict in a constructive way—even if the end result is the patients' decision to separate. The process of Positive Family Therapy acknowledges that this is a possibility.

The patient's concept is accepted, but counterconcepts are offered as a way to expand his conceptual horizon. The patient learns to see the relative nature of his own values. This relativization occurs in view of his own life history, the norms of his family, and the structure of his present situation. To arrive at this, we investigate positive aspects of infidelity, greed, pedantry, laziness, disorder, injustice, impudence, doubt, et cetera.

Lending Support to Self-help

In conjunction with the family members, the therapist works through their concepts: why it's hard for them to encourage their marriage partner (the problem of justice); why they are afraid of being rejected (trust); et cetera. In addition, we teach them the techniques of giving encouragement.

Encouraging Positive Traits

One must encourage positive traits, by saying things like "I find it fantastic that you didn't make me wait for you" and encourage the positive traits of discretionary behavior by saying things like "I used to think you were very impudent. But now I realize how well you make your point with other people and how little you are influenced by others. I, on the other hand, place a lot of weight on what others think." A further technique of the positive process is the two-sided criticism, where both recognition of the partner and one's honest reservations are given expression: "You are my model as far as career committment is concerned, but you have too little time for me" or "Granted, you don't have much time for me. But this gives me the chance to think about myself and develop my own interests."

The Psychoserum

One way to familiarize the patient with differentiated concepts and counterconcepts is the use of meditative preoccupation with him. In conjunction with relaxation training (autogenous training, progressive relaxation), in a tense moment—before falling asleep, for example—one envisions the concept and the counterconcept accompanying it. We call such an alternative concept a psychoserum. It is a formula-like abridgement of goals and meaningful ideas. It is designed to enable the patient to correct his conflict-laden behaviors and to strengthen a conscious impulse that in turn can make a behavioral change easier. Examples of the psychoserum are "Learn to distinguish between politeness and honesty" (for people who neglect their own interests out of sheer consideration of others); "Learn to distinguish between order and patience" (in the case of child-rearing difficulties that arise because of the child's messiness and the mother's pronounced demands for orderliness); "Learn to distinguish between love and justice" (for a patient who would like to avenge his wife's unfaithfulness), et cetera. (For further information, cf. Peseschkian, 1977).

GUIDELINES FOR SELF-HELP

Practice the Relativity of Values: Every individual has positive and negative qualities. Yet what is positive and what is negative is not absolutely certain, but depends on the concepts you use as your measurement. What you perceive as negative does not have to be seen the same way by your partner. Ask yourself which of your expectations and attitudes correspond to your critical behavior and that of your partner. With the aid of the tools of Positive Family Therapy, you can work out the critical behavioral areas.

Practice Situational Encouragement: Don't criticize your partner. Encourage him in his positive behavior for a week or two (in terms of content, briefly, and immediately). In this way, you will develop a foundation for trust in your relationship. It's not enough to conclude "You're a nice person" or "You have pretty eyes." It is more crucial that you strengthen a concrete form of behavior or an actual concept.

Practice Paradoxical Encouragement: Encourage your partner in his critical behavior as well. Look for the positive aspects that his "mistake" has for you and him. In this way your perspective will change. Previously you have mainly noticed your child's messiness, but now you also see a positive side to his messiness: his personal way of being messy and his creative association with it.

Work Through Your Resistance: For you, the question can be posed this way: "Why should I give encouragement to a marriage partner who angers me and whom I'd actually like to punish?" (justice). Try to answer this question for yourself.

Use a Psychoserum: Carry out autogenous training, progressive relaxation, or a different method of relaxing. When you feel marvelously relaxed, envision the positive aspects of the critical behavior. Example: "My depressions are segments of my getting rid of burdens. When I feel depressed, I let everything go—all my obligations, all my conformity, even myself. My depressions are a counterbalance to my need to always be the best and to do best" (said by a forty-three–year–old female patient).

Using Stories as Psychoserum: A large part of the concepts and counterconcepts have found expression in proverbs and stories. Their advantage is their malleable, lively form of expression. Imagine your concepts and counterconcepts in the form of stories and sayings: "We're not suited for each other. We are such completely different people" (concept). "Sameness calms us down. It's controvery that makes us productive" (counterconept).

4. The Stage of Verbalization

A REASON TO BE THANKFUL

"I need money. Can you lend me a hundred Tuman [Iranian currency]?" a man asked his friend.

"I have the money, but I won't give it to you. Be grateful for that!"

Angrily the friend replied, "That you have money and don't want to give it to me, I can rather understand. But that I should be grateful for it is not only incomprehensible, but a downright disgrace."

"My dear friend," the other answered, "you asked me for money. I could have said, 'Come tomorrow.' Tomorrow I would have said, 'I'm sorry I can't give it to you yet; come back the day after tomorrow.' If you had come to me then, I would have said, 'Come at the end of the week.' In this way I could have held you off till the end of time or at least until someone else had given you the money. But you wouldn't have found someone else, because you would have been so preoccupied with coming to me and you would have always counted on getting my money. So I tell you in all honesty that I am not going to give you the money. So you can look for it elsewhere and try to make your fortune there. Be grateful to me."

In the previous stages, we created the atmospheric requirement, opened up the rigid front a bit, and improved the patient's ability to understand. Now begins the direct confrontation in the family. One has expanded his own foundation by using the tools of Positive Family Therapy to develop a language for solving conflicts instead of carrying them out in a reactive way. Disturbed speech, which either completely avoids feelings or consists entirely of clichés, is the sign of a disturbance in one's interpersonal relationships.

Through the tools of Positive Family Therapy, the conflicts that had been carried out preverbally and unconsciously are now made concrete. In the therapeutic situation, we draw on a language in which everyday conflicts are formulated. But this time the language is used as a means of self-help and psychotherapy.

THERAPEUTIC FOCUS

Politeness—Honesty

The relationship between politeness and honesty is the key conflict at the level of verbalization. *Politeness* here means the recognition of conventional forms for interpersonal relationships, the neglect of one's own needs and interests in favor of others' needs and interests, and finally the obstruction of aggression because of social considerations: "I'm afraid to express my opinion because I don't want to lose the friendly opinions of other people." *Honesty*, on the other hand, means representing one's own interests—or adopting interests of one's own, as opposed to the interests of others: "I always express my opinion, regardless of whether other people like it or not." In order to grasp the conflict situation of the patient and his opportunities for communication, I look into his experiences and attitudes about politeness and honesty. I place them in a concrete situation and explore them through therapeutic conversation. In this way, communicative capabilities are developed and, at the same time, metacommunicative abilities are addressed. One learns to recognize disorders in interpersonal relationships, to understand their conditions and causes, to perceive the concepts and misunderstandings involved, and, where possible, to relieve the dissonance.

The therapist can address the family's basic conflict with reference to politeness—honesty and work out with them the specific meanings that *politeness* and *honesty* have for them. I ask concretely, "With whom and how often do conflicts about courtesty and honesty occur? How and when are they expressed? To what actual capabilities are they related?"

Differentiation analytical communication training in Positive Family Therapy can be applied in the one-on-one relationship of the patient and therapist, in family therapy, and in group therapy. In these latter cases, polite and honest behaviors can be tried out in an expanded social situation. For a self-check, these exercises can be presented to the family in role play or on video recorder.

In addition, the therapist tries to persuade the family to form a family group, parent group, partner group, et cetera.

GUIDELINES FOR SELF-HELP

Begin the Conversation: At this stage, speak about the conflicts and problems that are developing with your mate. Begin the conversation with encouragement.

Listen to Your Partner: You mate cites his problems and wishes. Listen carefully; be polite. Ask yourself and your mate what significance the problem has for him, for how long it has preoccupied him, and how he deals with it. Before you give any advice, try to learn to know his concept and to help him to experience and discover it as well. If he drinks, for example, what does this mean for him?

Be Honest: Make your own problems clear to your mate. How do you stand with them? What does the conflict mean for you? What would you like to achieve with it? What is your neuralgic point?

Look for Possible Solutions: Solutions that are feasible for both of you are sought. Remember that both you and your mate need time to take on a change of perspective. You have your own will, and so does your mate. If you have honestly said what you consider right, it's up to him to make of it what he wants. In reverse this is also true for you.

Follow Game Rules for the conversation: As far as the conversation is concerned, both people involved are obliged to keep quiet. But don't forget that blunt observations do more harm to you and your mate than does an open conversation conducted with care for your mate's feelings. Blunt observations are unfair to your partner. Don't just practice being critical. At the same time, say how it could be done better.

5. The Stage of Goal Expansion

A STORY ON THE WAY

Persian mysticism tells of a wanderer who trudged along on a seemingly endlessly long road. He was loaded down with all sorts of burdens. A heavy sack of sand hung on his back; a thick water hose was draped around his body. In his right hand, he carried an oddly shaped stone, in the left hand a boulder. Around his neck an old millstone dangled on a frayed rope. Rusty chains, with which he dragged heavy weights through the dusty sand, wound around his ankles. On his head, the man was balancing a half-rotten pumpkin. With every step he took, the chains rattled. Moaning and groaning, he moved forward step by step, complaining of his hard fate and the weariness that tormented him. On his way, a farmer met him in the glowing heat of midday. The farmer asked, "O tired wanderer, why do you load yourself down with this boulder?"

"Awfully dumb," replied the wanderer, "but I hadn't noticed it before." With that, he threw the rock away and felt much lighter.

Again, after going a long way down the road, a farmer met him and asked, "Tell me, tired wanderer, why do you trouble yourself with the half-rotten pumpking on your head, and why do you drag those heavy iron weights behind you on chains?"

The wanderer answered, "I'm very glad you pointed this out to me. I didn't realize what I was doing to myself." He took off the chains and smashed the pumpkin into the ditch alongside the road. Again he felt lighter. But the farther he went, the more he began to suffer again.

A farmer coming from the field watched him in amazement and said, "Oh good man, you are carrying sand in the sack, but what you see far off in the distance is more sand than you could ever carry. And your big water hose—as if you planned to cross the Kawir Desert. All the while there's a clear stream flowing alongside you, which will accompany you on your way for a long time." Upon hearing this, the wanderer tore open the water hose and emptied its brackish water onto the path. Then he filled a hole with the sand from his knapsack. He stood there pensively and looked into the sinking sun. The last rays sent their light to him. He glanced down at himself, saw the heavy millstone around his neck, and suddenly realized it was the stone that was still causing him to walk so bent over. He unloosened it and threw it as far as he could into the river. Freed from his burdens, he wandered on through the cool of the evening to find lodging.

A clever businessman does not put all his capital into one project. He divides it among several of them. Communication disorders usually bring with them a limitation of human contact. One punishes one's mate by forbidding him something, i.e., withdrawing from him. The results are a cooling off and a diminishment of the human relationships. We call this process the limitation of goals. The basic principle for goal expansion is the realization that our marriage partners possess a number of other potentials besides the areas that are conflictual.

THERAPEUTIC FOCUS

Goal expansion is the last stage in the five-phase process. In it there is a loosening of the psychotherapeutic relationship. It takes place under two aspects: the mourning work associated with the disaffiliation and, as a counter to it, the work on the patient's ability to develop activities for himself and to find pleasure in them. The previous stages, which all comprise elements of a goal expansion, provided the patient with the capacity for self-help. He is thus now better equipped to leave the therapeutic area and to turn to a form of self-help that can accompany him throughout his life. Goal expansion is oriented according to the neurotic restrictions of one's value fields, which usually concentrate on a few capabilities. But now the patient learns to shape his life anew and to keep goals in mind that he had pursued before his neurotic restrictions began and that had then been pushed into the background. More than anything else, the four areas for dealing with conflict are particularly suited as orientation aids for goal expansion.

The basis for goal expansion is the counterconcept, i.e., the expansion concept. Every lively encounter with a partner who has other concepts is already a potential goal expansion: What would you do if you didn't have problems? What wishes do you dream about? What would you do if you weren't a rational, sensible person? What can you learn from people who act differently than you?

Goal Expansion

Expand your goals in the area of the actual capabilities. (Which actual capabilities have you previously treated in a perfunctory manner?) Open up new ways for dealing with conflict. (Which areas have previously gotten the short end of things?) Which forms of relationships do you think can be developed between yourself and your partner (four model dimensions)?

Exchanging Roles

For one day, a partner should take over the role tasks of the other person. On another day, a particular member of the family, with his wishes and needs, can occupy the foreground. On another day, a different member has his "day." Finally, the family tries to figure out what needs and interests they have in common.

Familial, parental, and partner groups are continued. Not only do they contribute to overcoming problems, but they also open up new possibilities and goals for the future.

If The Partner Does Not Participate

What do you do if your partner won't go along with it? Remember that you have your own interests. You do not live for others, but for yourself. Frequently a partner needs a certain amount of time before he can accept your model. You should ask, "Why doesn't my partner want to participate?" This can uncover clues to misunderstandings: "Does he not want to participate because he feels caught unawares, or has he found a different way that I have trouble accepting?"

THE FIVE STAGES IN POSITIVE FAMILY THERAPY

If you do not help a man with his troubles, it is equivalent to bringing troubles to him.

—Oriental windom

The five-staged frame model is not a rigid pattern into which the patient and his family must be forced. The individual stages are not statically built on each other, but exist in a dynamic relationship with each other. During the whole therapeutic process there are moments that, in turn, lead to observation, discernment, encouragement, verbalization, and goal expansion. In an appropriate situation, they can become a focus for the treatment. On the other hand, each individual session contains the structure of the five phases. This is particularly true for the initial discussion in family therapy, when decisive impulses for activating the self-help can already be given. Here an essential goal of the treatment is already reached: The family works together on the foundation of the five stages in terms of self-help. The therapist is no longer the "leader" of the family group, but simply an "advisor." Often therapy is terminated after this initial discussion. What follows is self-help, and this lasts one's entire life.

FAMILY GROUP—PARENTAL AND PARTNER GROUP

Socialization and upbringing take place in the primary family, reeducation/therapy in the therapist-patient relationship, family group, parent group, partner group, or a group form that goes beyond the narrower family unit. Positive Family Therapy positions the family group against the background of other family activities. This sharp division occurs because it has been shown that family sessions isolated and limited in time can influence the family's daily life just as therapeutic sessions can have an impact on the patient's daily activities. The family group adheres to the game rules described below and uses the tools of Positive Family Therapy as aids in self-help.

The Family Group

All members of the family meet at a regular time that they all find agreeable. This can be on a weekly basis. But sessions can be called for special reasons. If one person can't come to a session because of unforeseen events and if the other members can be notified in time, a new time can be agreed upon. A family group session lasts from forty-five to sixty minutes. Sometimes the opportunity for the family group emerges automatically, as, for instance, after dinner, when the whole family is still sitting around the table. The terms "family group," "family council" (Dreikurs, 1973), or "family conference" (Gordon, 1972) do not need to be used at all. The informal summons to a discussion ("What do you think of our sitting down and talking about it?") frequently leads to creative and dynamic family sessions. Each member is accepted as an equal partner.

The Group Journal

Each member writes down in his own notebook the topics he'd like to propose, as well as agreements and decisions reached by the group as a whole. Only in the family group is there criticism. Until then, observations are written down in the group notebook.

But memory for good intentions seems even weaker than memory for experiences. Here the note card can be a big help. Often simply grabbing for the note card marked "Politeness" can prevent insulting a partner or hurting his feelings. The note card labeled "Orderliness" reminds one that aggravation can be avoided by adopting a more careful behavior.

At the agreed time, the family group meets and, if possible, sits in a circle around a table. It is important that no one sits too far from the others. It is best that the T.V., radio, and other disturbing influences be turned off. But even there, agreement from the entire group should be obtained first. Wait until everyone is there. The first topic of discussion is the successes of individual family members, the solutions to problems, and pleasant events. Along with fulfilling other functions, this form of positive introduction confirms the group goals that have been accomplished and recognizes them within the family community. Then the family group turns to problems, conflicts, and wishes. The group assistant, who is chosen before each session, asks, "Who would like to say something today? Who has a particular problem?" The problems brought up are gathered and worked through. The group assistant asks each member for his opinion of the problems, focusing on the following questions: What is the problem?; What are the causes, backgrounds, concepts, goals and interests hidden behind the problem?; and What possible solutions exist? All members of the family, particularly the parents, are given the task of searching for the positive aspects of the conflict under discussion.

The theme that has the greatest significance for this particular group session becomes the motto of the week. Thus there is a "Politeness Week," "Orderliness Week," "Honesty Week," "Punctuality Week," et cetera.

Distribution of Functions and Exchange of Roles

The distribution of functions can be regarded as a basic principle in the family group. Only when a partner can share in another's problems is it possible for him to understand that person. Frequently, a rigid division of roles in the family prevents the parents from gaining insight into their children's problems, and vice versa. The exchange of roles is the most direct way of shaping the family structure in a dynamic way. For a limited time, a member of the group takes over tasks and role characteristics that had previously been assigned to another person. The father, for instance, acts as the housewife, the mother takes over responsibility for making plans that the father had taken care of, and the children, for their part, take on tasks and functions that had been part of the parental responsibility, e.g. household planning and advising.

Significance of the Family Group

Current problems are not the only ones that are discussed in the family group. Plans are also made for future undertakings—purchases, trips, inviting company over, parties, gifts. Every member of the family thus learns to work actively in the family and becomes aware that the family group is not just formal arrangement or the source of problems, but that he can exert influence on the family's decisions. Within the family, which to a certain extent functions without conscious control, there is usually an unconscious division of roles, strongly held disinclinations, and particular preferences. Since a family group functions simultaneously, i.e., with all members present at the same time and actively participating in the group, there is a move toward many-sided and -leveled transfers and emotional involvements. These can help to better control the ties and conflicts.

Just as the total flavor of a casserole cannot be traced to a single ingredient, so also attitudes, behavioral patterns, and decisions in a group cannot be exclusively traced back to an individual or to a few family members. Rather, it is the work of the entire group.

The family group as we have presented it here is an ideal typical family group, a target value. The actual group event can be oriented according to this formal guide. Since feelings cannot be arranged very easily, this presentation of the family group was intentionally limited to specific game rules. But at least equally important are the emotional atmosphere in which the family event is carried out and the mutual understanding and the willingness to empathize with the other family members, even when one has conflicts with them. According to my experiences, stubborn tensions in the family can be objectivized and broken down if, for example, stories are told within the family group that are relevant to the existing problems. The story frequently becomes a central pole around which the subsequent discussion revolves. In the same way, the tools of Positive Family Therapy can be presented at such a group session and can then be worked through. In so doing, it has been verified that everyone answers these questions.

Parental and Partner Group

Regarding the problems that concern the children, the parents should—at least in principle—be united in front of the family group. Otherwise, it is suggested that the parents set aside a certain time—for example, the evening—to discuss their disagreements. In this way they can deal with the problem early enough but not draw the children into the conflicts.

Such a parent session should not last longer then fifteen to thirty minutses. It is better to talk for fifteen minutes every evening, if possible, than once a month till midnight. As an aid, the Differentiation Analytical Inventory can also be used. In its structure and techniques, the parent group is modelled on the partner group.

Maxims for the Parent Group

A good partnership is not one where there are no problems and conflicts, but one where there is a willingness to discuss them openly and matter-of-factly and to work them through. A partnership is no insurance agency. It is, rather, a balancing act between love and justice.

Couples can learn to discuss problems from various areas of life (like child rearing, problems at work, large plans and tasks, sexual problems, conflicts with in-laws and acquaintances). If one has the feeling he can't deal with the marital problems by himself or if the problem concerns the relationships only secondarily (e.g., intense jealousy about the partner's earlier sexual experiences), it is advisable to secure the advice of a specialist.

Conflicts tend to proliferate like malignant tumors and to penetrate areas that at first seem to have been untouched. The partner group can work to counter this tendency. Conflicts can be limited by temporal and spatial barriers and can be treated by the partners involved. The procedures in the partner group correspond in principle to the methodology we have already met in the family group. It presents the members with an undoubedly difficult task, which makes it seem to some people that they must constantly try to jump over their own shadow. Actually, it is not easy to suddenly start up conversations with a mate whom one has been punishing with silence. It is not easy to establish distance from one's customary forms of exchange. Often enough, such an adjustment is accompanied by a loss of status. Occasionally, the role divisions in the marital rlelationship become unsure. To help counter these difficulties, the self-help phases are available: observation/distancing, inventory, situational encouragement, verbalization, and goal expansion.

Questions That every Partner Should Ask Him/herself in the Marital Conflict Situation

Can the problem be solved?
Do I want to really change anything?
Can my partner come up to my expectations?
Does he/she want a solution to the problem?
Have I already attempted to find a solution?
Do I see our situation honestly and openly?
Do I express my opinion in an honest way?
Am I ready to listn to my partner, too?
Am I really ready to give my partner time and to take time myself?
Do I expect changes to take place from one minute to the next?
Do I expect the other person to change, and am I ready for change msyself?
Am I still giving myself and my partner a chance?
Do I stick with my partner even during a major conflict?
If we can't handle our problems alone, are we willing to seek help from a specialist?

6. The Strategy of Positive Family Therapy

If one is cruel to himself, how can we expect him to be compassionate with others?

—Oriental wisdom

The following strategies of Positive Family Therapy present an overview of the applicational possibilities of its tools. They are flexibly adapted to the specific needs of the situation in which the patient or patient family happens to be. The strategies outlined here, as my colleagues and I have found in our own experiences with Positive Family Therapy, have proved themselves to be advantageous. They are the result of discussions with patient families and critical talks among colleagues. In the following sections, I present some typical constellations and images of illness where definite behaviors exist. The following parameters should be given attention:

1. The way the patient or family presents itself for the therapy: individual patient, nuclear family, extended family, therapy in opposition to the family, as "Therapy without a Patient."
2. The image of the illness that the patient or family produces: Here it is mainly a question of how much stress the patient or family can take, what its capacity is. It has proved to be worthwhile to orient oneself according to a distinction between neurotic, psychosomatic, and psychotic patients. Each of these patient groups requires its own approach.
3. Possible or desired length of treatment: Particular situations require a flexible approach to the length of the treatment. In practice, this means the shorter the actual therapeutic intervention can be, the more emphasis must be placed on the aspect of self-help. In an extreme case, this means that the patient family is familiarized with the tools of Positive Family Therapy and the therapist simply supervises the self-help activities that then ensue. The situation occurs with families that have

good resources for self-help, with families where external circumstances limit the length of the treatment, and with patients whose treatment takes place within a set length of time, e.g., during a stay in a sanitarium.

4. The focus for dealing with conflict: Since families already have some self-help activities at their disposal, the treatment does not have to begin at a therapeutic zero. Instead, it is important that one become sensitive to the self-help mechanisms that are already being used. Therapeutically, this means placing emphasis on areas that had previously been blocked off. At this point, the Positive Process is used in a concrete way.

THE NUCLEAR FAMILY (FATHER—MOTHER—CHILDREN)

The central problem is the relationship "Connectedness—Differentiation—Detachment" as stages of the child-parent relationship. In terms of content, these three forms of interaction are related to the actual capabilities. Since the parents are primarily the transmitters of self-help, we work through the four model-dimensions with them, taking into consideration both their own role as models as well as their relationships to their own parents. In connection with the actual capabilities and the four forms for dealing with conflict, we investigate the parents' marital problems. The primary focus of the self-help is the first stage: observation/distancing. We found again and again that a successful first stage is the prerequisite for the other four stages. In some cases, the parents can be brought into group therapy with other parents. But one can also consider individual therapy appropriate to the existing problem. From the viewpoint of a social model situation with children of the same age (goal expansion), the child can be placed in a therapeutic children's group. Here it has proved to be valuable to carry out games (role playing, projected transference of one's own conflicts, et cetera) in connection with stories.

CRISIS INTERVENTION

With severe family problems, it is essential that the basic capabilities be activated in the individual and his partner. If the partnership is in danger of dissolving, it has been advisable not to persist with the existing problems, but to start by speaking to the self-help activities and by assigning the partner the five stages of Positive Family Therapy. Only later do we return to the conflicts and an analysis of their contents. We look into the symptoms, giving them a positive interpretation, and try to make possible an alternative system of relationships to the problem. Because of rigid communication structures, the stage of verbalization is put into the therapeutic situation, with the therapist working to equalize differences, make discoveries, and provide new interpretations. Within the framework of self-help, the stages of observation/distancing, situational encouragement, and goal expansion are placed in the foreground.

MARITAL PROBLEMS

Here the complaints usually deal with situations surrounding the actual capabilities. We deal with this in a therapeutic way and begin with the actual capabilities (DAI). The next step consists in rethinking the symptoms or the critical actual capabilities in a positive way, whereby we can also make use of transcultural examples. In order to make mutual understanding easier, the four model dimensions become the theme. After the first session, the following procedure has proved to be practical: The cooperative partner—sometimes it is the partner who has more time—takes over the role of therapist and, under supervision, carries out the first three stages. Only after creating the necessary prerequisites for communication in this way, does the actual partner therapy begin (at the stage of verbalization and goal expansion).

PSYCHOSOMATICS AND THE FAMILY

The distinguishing mark of many psychosomatic patients is the denial of conflict, which often appears as an ignoring of family conflicts. The task is to get from the psychosomatic symptom to the psychosocial conflicts they are based on, and from there to actually dealing with the conflict.

The starting point for the treatment is the four areas for dealing with conflict. They are particularly suited for this because psychosomatic patients usually present themselves with their symptoms. From the forms for dealing with conflict, we move on to the microtraumas (actual capabilities [DAI]). Only then do we speak to the basic conflict in the form of the four model dimensions. A key role in all this is the positive interpretation of the symptoms, which should preferably come from the patient himself. He knows the significance that his illness has had in his life—often, indeed, he knows it more than anyone.

Depending on the situation, the patient himself can take on an active role in the five stages of self-help. In some cases, a different member of the family takes on this task. Of course, in the five stages, the first stage is the first to be taken up. Here the crucial thing is not to observe the symptoms but the conditions under which they occur. The stage of inventory helps lead to a differentiated way of looking at things. At the stage of verbalization, the conflict theme politeness-honesty has proven to be a key conflict for psychosomatic patients.

PSYCHOSES IN POSITIVE FAMILY THERAPY

Here I have in mind acute situations or those where there is a danger of decompensation. In general, those principles are valid that have already been pointed out for working with the nuclear family. For the therapist and the patient family, the first step is the positive interpretation of the symptoms, i.e., pointing out the function the symptoms have for the family. The four forms for dealing with conflict are an aid in this process. How do a schizophrenic and his family members work out the problems they have in common? Much as in a marital crisis, the basic capabilities are the basis for the treatment. Together with the patient family, the actual capabilities (DAI) and the four model dimensions are worked through. In doing so, it is important to clarify the preconscious concepts. The goal is that the family members first learn to accept the deviant behavior and to understand its positive value (e.g., to distance themselves from the concept "What will people say?") Another goal is to speak directly to the capabilities that are intact in the patient and his family. To avoid decompensation, the process is not one of discovery, but is primarily directed toward ego support. This goal is aided by the positive interpretation, as well as by stories that can help give the family a change of perspective. For the family members, the focus lies first of all in taking inventory of personal perception and attitudinal patterns and then in situational encouragement. For the patient, the emphasis is on a goal expansion that is oriented toward the stage of inventory. With patients whose symptoms are socially conspicuous, family treatment is often not enough. We are left with no other choice but to bring in other groups (teachers, perhaps colleagues, the treating physician, social workers, et cetera).

EXTENDED FAMILY THERAPY

This can include relatives (parents, siblings, uncles, aunts, grandparents, in-laws, et cetera) as well as other people who for some reason have an important function for the family (good friends, teachers, the family doctor, et cetera). Therapy of family groups of this kind can be conducted in the form of one or several sessions together. This procuedure has been particularly effective when the existing conflicts appeared as problems of the extended family or when conflictual concept traditions and delegations occupied the foreground. The concept family tree can be worked out via the concepts (oriented to the forms for dealing with conflict, the four model dimensions, the DAI, and the interaction stages). This thematic structuring of the therapeutic work with the extended family makes it possible to proceed in a differentiated way and to avoid the confusion with which a large family group is used to reacting to generalized conflicts.

FAMILY THERAPY WITHOUT THE PARTNER

Under this rubric, there is a multitude of life situations that contain a family problem, but where the spouse and/or other family members either do not want to or cannot take part in the treatment. In practice, this is treatment of the individual patient. The family, though, appears in the DAI in the way the patient experiences it. Although the treatment situation is individual, family therapy activities come to the fore in the self-help part of therapy. The patient carries out the five stages of self-help in his family or partnership and is controlled by therapeutic supervision. If the patient has no family at this point of the treatment and is still socially isolated, the five stages can be applied to relationships with other conflict partners (e.g., to the service personnel at the clinic, to colleagues, and also, in one's imagination, to members of one's original family). One determines, for instance, which actual capabilities became conflict potentials, how the four model dimensions came into the picture, which concepts were involved, et cetera. In view of the verbalization stage, the therapist can at this point become a functional substitute for the family. The detachment then occurs as the stage of goal expansion where the imagined, fantasized possibilities breached by the therapist, patient, or group relationship are now led over into social reality. Correspondingly, the emphasis here is on goal expansion, the stage for which all the other stages and the positive interpretation were the foundation.

POSITIVE GROUP PSYCHOTHERAPY

Positive Family Therapy works in a way that is concentrated on themes. The themes to be discussed (e.g., fidelity in connection with marital problems) or are presented by the therapist in the form of stories. These stories then provide forms of association for the group members. An important structural principle for group psychotherapy is the three interaction stages: connectedness —differentiation —detachment. Within these categories, the tools of Positive Family Therapy are worked through step by step. Hence for a considerable period of time the actual capabilities, the four forms for dealing with conflict, et cetera can become the thematic center of the group. The emphasis, however, is not on the acquisition of a theoretical competence. Rather, the goal is that within the group each member remembers his personal experiences and concepts in connection with the theme at hand. To extend this information, the therapist expands the group's concepts through, for example, alternative transcultural concepts. Positive reinterpretations help overcome crises in the group. But this does not necessarily mean that one intervenes in a placating or appeasing manner. Instead, the group members get new information through the positive reinterpretation, and this information can stimulate them to find new solutions and strategies for the individual member.

POSITIVE SELF-HELP GROUPS

What we have said about group psychotherapy is technically valid. But in the self-help group, the emphasis is on the actual conflict. In connection with the German Association for Positive Psychotherapy (DGPP), teachers' groups, lawyers' groups, and physicians' groups have been formed as self-help groups to deal with the special problems of their particular profession. The essential thing here is self-discovery, a new awareness of one's own concepts and feelings. The members of the self-discovery groups use the instruments of Positive Family Therapy to recognize and learn about their own concepts and to relate them in the group by means of transcultural, interdisciplinary examples. The positive self-help group points in three directions:

1. At such relationships as physician-patient, teacher-pupil, lawyer-client, et cetera;
2. At the relationship of physicians (or lawyers, teachers, et cetera) to their colleagues and, beyond that, the possibility for working cooperatively on interdisciplinary issues;
3. At the relationship of the participant to his own family.

This form of self-help group is conceived to be a step toward a more comprehensive community psychology where it is possible for representatives of various disciplines to work together, to take a more extensive view of psychohygienic considerations, and to make use of their skills as humans and colleagues in the process of self-help.

7. The Relationships between Therapeutic Models

Since neurotic, psychotic, and psychosomatic disorders can be viewed as a diminishments of one's connections with reality, the four forms for deaing with conflict become the therapeutic guideline. We can differentiate between forms that are hypertrophic, highly differentiated, and perfectly imbalanced, on the one hand, and, on the other hand, those forms that became conflict potentials by virtue of the fact that they lacked opportunities for development. In other words, a person can become ill not only from what he has experienced, but also from what he was unable to experience when the necessary developmental conditions were removed from the capabilities inherent in man. Both conflict dispositions develop cumulatively as the almost unnoticed accumulation of microtraumas that correspond to the social concepts existing in the family and processed by it. As a result, we depict the four forms for dealing with conflict in two corresponding, complementary pictures.

The Four Forms for Dealing with Conflict as the Expression of Overemphasis and Overdifferentiation

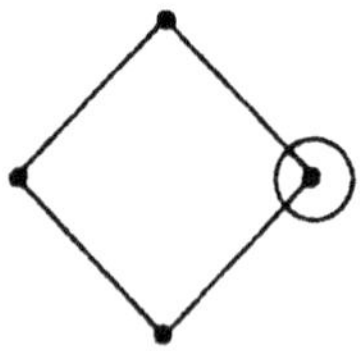

Achievement

The Four Forms for Dealing with Conflict as the Expression of Areas That Have Been Overshadowed

Body

Fantasy

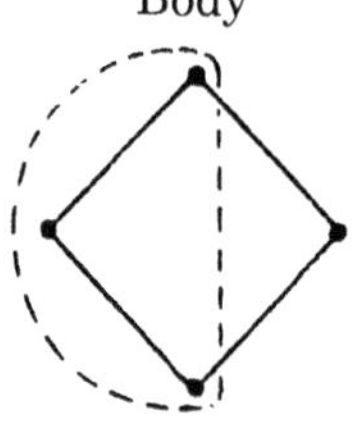

Contact

This diagram describes a typical form of conflict susceptibility that becomes accessible in terms of life history by means of the four model dimensions; in addition, its contents are described through the Differentiation Analytical Inventory. The functional relationships of the models can be illucidated with this pithy example: A thirty-four–year–old businessman came to my practice after many years of attempted treatment with other therapists. Most of all, he felt he had to present a good image. He was suffering from functional heart trouble, repeated stomach pains, and feelings of anxiety—particularly the fear of failure. His previous therapy had dealt mostly with psychosomatic processes and the achievement problems associated with his career. Following the models presented, we expanded the therapeutic spectrum: In the foreground of the problem was achievement as the form for dealing with conflict. For as long as he could remember, his life had revolved around achievement. The ideal image he made of himself focused on the concepts of success and his ability to be actively advancing and unyielding to compromise. This narcissistic desire for unattainable perfection went hand in hand with an intense fear of failure. Negative variances in his repertoire for dealing with conflict are in these areas: BODY, CONTACT, AND FANTASY. Although they had contributed much to the dynamics of his conflict, the patient was unaware of them. For him, they stood at the edge of his reality and were no longer a source of joy; they remained deficient and, for their part, produced further anxieties. But they are comprehensible against the background of the four model dimensions that describe the family relationships he had originally experienced. These anxieties proved to be a fear of loss of object. Achievement had been adopted as a delegation task. In view of the achievement problem, the patient had entered into a fusion with the paternal image. On the other hand, the deficient areas pointed to the patient's potential need, a need expressed—viewed teleologically—as a formation of symptoms. Both parents worked and were active, enabling him to acquire their emotional attention only through his activity and achievement. To a large part, contact was limited to the immediate family. When they did go beyond the confines of the family, it was for business purposes. Other forms of contact were "dumb" or were avoided, if at all possible, because the family feared a possible rivalry. But in contrast to this there developed an ideal figure, a comrade who would stand by the patient even if things were going bad for him or when he wasn't capable of being such an achiever. But, at the same time, the patient remained critical of this ideal, because he feared a comrade like that did not exist and that his desire to lean on someone would damage his independence and his resistance to compromise.

Achievement was occupied in a compensatory, narcissistic way. It was the area where the patient could find confirmation of his desire for a grandiose self. In regard to his own body "I," to interpersonal contacts, and to fantasies that were not concerned with achievement, there was an almost unavoidable need. In this area he proved to be particularly sickly.

For his own protection, he created in his fantasies a grandiose comrade who would never disappoint him and who—like a good father—would tolerate it when the patient revealed himself to be weak or unable to accomplish something. But such a fantasy was repudiated as being unrealistic, and the patient gave up any effort to establish a real and durable relationship. After all, no one could come up to his fantastic ideal and meet his expectations and demands.

Among the actual capabilities, industry/achievement, thrift, orderliness, punctuality, and reliability were in the foreground. They occur again in the concepts that were expressed in the patient's lifestyle. He referred to them as the motivating forces that stamped the situation of his upbringing.

The conflict situation can be described as follows:

Forms for Healing with Conflict (Overemphasized Areas)	Four Model Dimensions (Development of the Concepts of Self and Society)	Forms for Dealing with Conflict (Non-experienced Areas)

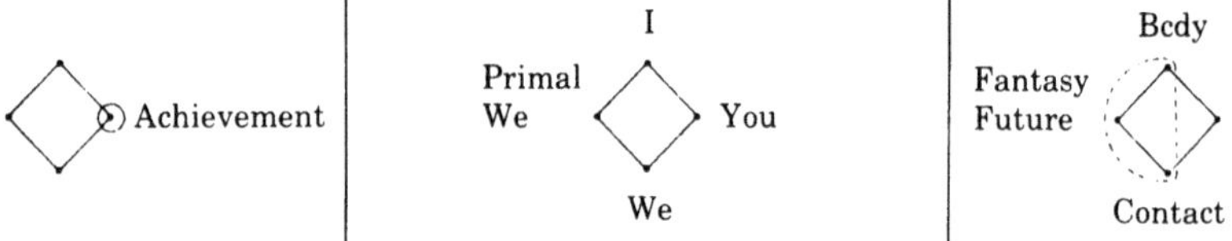

Overemphasis on Achievement (Fear of Failure)

Actual Capability	I	mother	father
Industry/ achievement	+ +	+ +	+ +
thrift	+ +	+ +	+ +
orderliness	+ +	+ +	+ +
punctuality	+ + +	+ +	+ + +
reliability	+ +	+ +	+ +
contact	–	–	–

Actual Capabilities from the DAI

The therapeutic strategy is directed primarily at the nonexperienced areas, which can be reworked in the sense of a reeducation (goal expansion in view of the body "I," interpersonal relationships, and the activities of fantasy. Going hand in hand with this is the autobiographical analysis of the overemphasized areas, the backgrounds to which become transparent to the patient.

8. Positive Family Therapy: Language and Social Strata

The talk of the child in the street is that of his father or mother at home.

—Oriental wisdom

It is considered a platitude that the customary forms of psychotherapy—primarily its chief exponent, psychoanalysis—prefer their patients to be from the upper and middle classes. This may be due to the fact that psychotherapists generally come from these classes themselves (Fromm, 1979). Since the psychotherapists' forte is intensive personal relationship—relationships that are easier to develop if the parties involved "speak the same language"—there is almost automatically an unspoken choice of patients. Furthermore, the techniques of customary psychotherapy, insofar as they view themselves as "revealing psychotherapies," require a typical form of differentiated speech behavior. In doing so, they exclude a number of potential patients from psychotherapy, labeling them as "unproductive patients."

A reason for this can be found in the language forms that sociolinguists have attributed to certain social classes (Bernstein, 1963; Oevermann, 1972). According to these findings, the middle class is characterized by its socioeconomic features and by its emphatic attention to the ability to express oneself verbally. This corresponds to their educational style, whereby the child's behavior is geared toward the feelings of the other person, i.e., to the consequences of particular actions, as when the parent says, "Daddy will be happy, disappointed, angry, delighted. . . . Daddy will be unhappy if you keep doing that." These appeals, usually carried out under threats that the parent will withdraw his love (Bernstein, 1964), arouse a sense of guilt in the child: "The child learns to deal with interpersonal tensions by learning to endure his guilt feelings and by using language to become aware of the consequences of his actions" (p. 92). Bernstein calls this differentiated language from the "elaborated code." His ideas approach those of the usual psychotherapies, which build the therapeutic relationship in a similar way by using the medium of language.

The members of the lower working class—so Bernstein asserts—do not have a command of the communication forms and sensibilities necessary for a psychotherapeutic relationship—not out of an inherent lack of intelligence, of course, but because of culturally determined systems of communication. As a result, a patient from the lower social classes has no orientation for therapeutic relationships (1964, p. 84). Bernstein shows that these people probably derive less benefit from therapy and terminate it earlier, while the therapist finds that the treatment is not rewarding for him either. According to sociologists, these problems in understanding are caused by the "limited code" that gives the speaker a speech model where little differentiation is possible. The language tends to be directive, as in such examples as "Clean up your room," "Stop that," and "At your age, people don't do that anymore." These status-oriented appeals are related to general rules associated with families or are dependent on particular positions. And these rules guide one's behavior: "Status appeals are impersonal. To be effective, they rely on the status of the person involved. Their goal is to perpetuate the culture or local traditions by increasing the similarity between the group and the person in question. If a child rebels, he challenges immediately the culture he belongs to. The culture thus tends to exert force on the individual, threatening him with punishment" (Bernstein, 1964, p. 91): "We were all industrious and decent people. A loafer like you won't get anywhere with us."

The appeals of the restricted code usually take place in an averbal context. The sentence "Do that" is not expressed in language, but by means of a gesture signifying, for instance, that the person should do the dishes. Mimetic expressions, rolling one's eyes, or a tone of irritation in the speaking voice clearly indicate a command or request.

The elaborated code that is typical of the middle class would approach this situation differently. One would try to explain why the person should do the dishes, why the speaker does not have time to do it himself, and how the whole family would benefit from it. And finally, the speaker would express his displeasure if the order is not followed: "You aren't a bit of help around here. You don't think of anyone but yourself. Since you won't help me, you'll have to take care of your own things from now on."

But most of all, the restricted code can develop within the family, thus proving to be sufficient to convey understanding within that small group. In the family, the members play by rules that, while conveying a feeling of community, actually have little to do with verbal processes.

In particular areas, members of the middle and upper classes likewise demonstrate a "restricted" language like that attributed to the lower class. But these areas are blind spots that remain undifferentiated against the background of the family and individual history: "My husband claims he's from a better class of people than I, but he is not able to talk about the problems in our relationship. He just says I'm imagining things. But on the other hand, he can get up at meetings at work and talk about organizational problems for hours on end." This quote from a thirty-one–year–old college teacher, married to a businessman, shows that *the problem of the "restricted code" in psychotherapy thus has a general significance for people of all classes.*

It takes on particular importance in connection with psychosomatic illnesses. It has been shown that psychosomatic patients, i.e., those who react to mental conflicts with physical symptoms, likewise have limited use of speech (S. Stephanos, 1973). Even when they are able to verbalize things in their daily lives, they can't seem to talk about their feelings and their inner lives. They lack the expressive capabilities for that, and to make up for it, they use body language. This group, too, tends to be treated shabbily by traditional psychotherapy. Psychotherapy tends to require verbal abilities and therefore prefers to treat neurotic patients. Psychotherapy shuts itself off from psychosomatic patients who are not as skilled at verbalization.

Positive Family Therapy tries to overcome these psychotherapeutic language barriers. The following theses outline the principles of Positive Family Therapy that will be discussed more fully in later parts of this book:

1. The therapeutic situation in family therapy allows the patient to remain in his customary communicative realm. As a "temporary member of the family," the therapist can grasp those things contained in the family's code and can ask the members to explain them. In this way, the therapist encourages the development of verbal differentiation. The ability to verbalize a conflict is not considered a prerequisite for treatment. On the contrary, Positive Family Therapy makes it possible for the family members to acquire this skill.
2. Even if language styles differe among the various social classes, the contents of their conflicts nevertheless remain comparable. Sears, Maccoby, and Levin (1957) found that working-class mothers displayed much stricter demands that their children adapt and accede to the prevailing order than did middle-class mothers. The working class mothers also inforced these expectations more strictly. Bernstein (1959) and Thomas

(1972) confirmed this tendency in extensive studies. Particular contents in child rearing and in conflicts thus appear to have a general significance, even if they are carried out in differentiated educational styles. In Positive Family Therapy, we make these contents the thematic center of the treatment. As "actual capabilities," they are easily comprehended, provide entry into the particular problem regardless of the social class, and are well suited to show the interaction with the relational systems operating in the society.

3. The tools of Positive Family Therapy give the patient access to his inherent ability to deal with his problems. They also enable him to develop the linguistic ability to come to terms with his feelings. The tools of Positive Psychotherapy thus establish the basis for a therapeutic intervention. This is particularly true for psychosomatic patients whose awareness of their problems is fostered by the tools themselves. It helps to take the "psychosomatic," who is entangled in his feelings, and convert him into a "neurotic," one who can perceive his conflicts on the level of contradictory feelings.
4. The process of verbalization requires verbal abstractions. One must first tackle the difficult job of gaining access to the fantasy by means of verbal forms. This is why Positive Family Therapy offers the patient stories, parables, sayings, and examples from other situations and cultures. They help him make associations that, like a therapeutic bridge, enable him to reveal his own existing conflicts. This also helps dismantle some of the misgivings about traditional therapy. The tormented silence that keeps many verbally undifferentiated, inhibited, and "unproductive" patients away from psychotherapy is avoided by these therapeutic means.

An additional aspect of Positive Family Therapy extends its applicability in terms of the language barriers. The therapy systematically develops within its therapeutic program particular measures that can be used in self-help. This enables the patient to play an active role in his own situation. It reduces the risk of excessive dependence on his therapist and leads him to master his situation.

Part VII.

Practice of Positive Family Therapy

1. Concepts and Their Application in Positive Family Therapy

A teacher's work is like that of a gardener who takes care of various plants. One plant loves the sunshine, the other the cool shade; one loves the shore of the stream, the other the barren mountain peak. One thrives in sandy soil, the other in rich loam. Each requires the care best suited for it; otherwise the result is unsatisfactory.

—Abdu'l 'Bahá

Previously, family therapy dealt mainly with problems of role divisions, family dynamics, family structures, and communications. The content of the dealings that took place between family members was usually eliminated from the theoretical considerations. Of course the therapist dealt with the aspect of contents, but merely as an accompanying phenomenon of the dynamic orientation.

I try to grasp the contents of the conflict as well as its dynamics and to make them useful for the therapy. These contents describe programs and qualities of interpersonal relationships that have taken shape as attitudes, values, and norms.

An example of this can be seen in a family of three people. For the father, it is important that punctuality and orderliness predominate. His wife's and children's messiness upsets him. But he isn't as fussy when it comes to honesty in his married life. He imagines how it would be to have a mistress; it wouldn't be at all hard for him to justify his behavior. The wife is the epitome of neatness and cleanliness. She can't stand to see a speck of dust on the furniture. Politeness is also important to her. If her child doesn't greet a visitor with a proper "hello," the mother gets upset. She thinks that complete honesty and fidelity, with no deviations are the foundation for every marriage. This bit of information about the contents of the family already sketches some essential conflict potentials in the family situation. The game rules contained in these descriptions take shape in the consciousness, behavior, and perceptions of the family (or group) members as they face specific concepts. We thus see a network of concepts that correspond to the personality structures of the family members and to the transaction structures of the family itself.

ACTUAL CONCEPTS AND BASIC CONCEPTS

Conflict situations can be described as confrontations between divergent values. As attitudes and behavioral patterns, these values are relatively stable. But not all concepts are equally important for the person's life plan or for the structure of a group. They influence behavior and feelings to various degrees. This is why we differentiate between various degrees of determination among the concepts.

Actual concepts (situational concepts) are direct motives for behavior and are influenced mainly by situational factors. A situational concept of this type can be seen in the complaints of a woman whose husband shows no intention of straightening up his things in the living room: "My husband's mess is getting on my nerves." This assertion says something about the man as well as about the woman who expresses this opinion.

Basic concepts (concepts linked to the personality) are repeated, often without detriment to the situation in which they are realized. One acts in a personal, unchanging style. He observes the game rules that he is used to living by. He can't easily abandon them in a particular situation, even if they prove to be hazardous or difficult for him to maintain. Concepts, indeed, play a game of hide-and-go-seek. From the outside, one cannot see how closely they are linked with the experiences, actions, and self-esteem of the individual. In this sense, a situational concept can contain symptomatic traits of the basic conflict. Behind apparently superficial utterances, there is all too often a statement that closely touches the ego. The woman's complaint about her husband's messiness can thus include a different nuance and can point to concepts associated with the personality. The phrase "Orderliness is half of life" goes into operation here with all its meaning. In its terse form, this sentence reflects a basic concept that covers a wide range of behaviors and comprises the person's total system. In this case, the sentence "Orderliness is half of life" becomes a concept that determines the behavior of a person and his expectations regarding himself and other people. We can describe this process as generalizing.

The generalizing associated with such a concept goes even further. Someone who lives by the optimistic phrase "Take it easy" has other ways of dealing with conflict than does a person who reacts to both success and failure with a resigned "What difference does it make?" The basic conflict describes both the cognitive and emotional structures according to which a person reacts to conflict. In a condensed form, it reflects the basic conflict: the learning that took place in the individual's past, the traditions he has adopted, the "collective and individual mythology." The term "individual mythology" is understood to refer to the concepts as crystallization of the attitudes of the individual. The collective mythology, on the other hand, comprises concepts that are detached from the individual and have acquired a social reality in communication and tradition.

All of us have such mythologies at our disposal, as well as consciously controlled concepts and more comprehensive relational systems that determine our possibilities. To put it in more general terms, every behavior and every attitude stands within the framework of basic concepts.

2. Concepts in Therapeutic Work: The Change of Perspective

"Tree, if you had changed your place in time, you would not have had to experience the hardness of the ax or the sharpness of the saw."

—Saadi

A typical characteristic of mental, psychosomatic, and psychosocial disorders is the imbalance of the concepts and the rigidity with which one clings to them. One's own concepts are defended as well as possible against the threats that come from other attitudes and concepts. It becomes an explosive situation not only when situational concepts are called into question, but also when one feels that those concepts that guarantee an important balance in the family are threatened. The concepts are joined by the apparent inability to accept deviations from the concepts. This emphasis on concepts can be illustrated with an example from brain research.

Cats were divided into two groups, one allowed to see only vertical and the other only horizontal lines in the first weeks of life. Subsequently, these cats were "blind" to lines on the plane other than the one they had viewed in early life. Surrounded by vertical lines, the "horizontal" animals began to stagger and lose their balance. The same thing happened when "vertical cats" were placed in a horizonal environment. This experiment (cf. Vester, 1978) can be compared to the situation of a person who grew up with a certain conceptual pattern and now finds himself in a group that has other concepts; he has lost his orientation. Someone who has learned a certain behavioral form (politeness) in his family and then adopted it for himself usually has trouble dealing with a situation where other rules of courtesy predominate and where he has to adjust his own program for politeness. If he doesn't have sufficient possibilities for making this adjustment, there can develop group problems or problems of self-esteem.

The initial goal of the therapeutic process is to loosen the rigidity and present the patient and his family with other possibilities. The technique that can be used here is the change of perspective. It can be facilitated by a positive interpretation of the concepts.

The positive process means that one becomes aware of the relativity of the concepts and comes to realize that a different, even contradictory concept does not provide a threat but an expansion of his horizon. This can be achieved by changing one's point of view: one learns to define the conflictual game rules in new ways and thereby finds new approaches and possible solutions.

The purpose of psychotherapy is not to replace one fixed concept with an equally fixed concept from an authoritarian therapist. The therapist can only try to differentiate the patient's concepts, his individual mythology, and then point out alternative concepts. The question of what's right and wrong is superseded by the question of what leads to which results and what preconditions set the stage for a particular mythology. Therapeutic concepts have a hypothetical character about them. The patient can accept them on a test basis and apply them to appropriate situations. By asking questions about the concept, we shine a light on otherwise unconscious, stereotypical relationships that are taken for granted—relational systems that determine how a person perceives his reality.

The willingness to change one's point of view sometimes leads to a chaotic situation where the identity associated with the concepts is called into question. This is why we do not bring about changes in perspective with a technique akin to alternating between hot and cold baths. It is precisely this approach that is facilitated by using Middle Eastern stories as a part of Positive Family Therapy.

3. Stories and Sayings as Aids for Changing One's Perspective

One shouldn't throw old habits out the window, but should politely escort them to the front door.

—Oriental wisdom

Positive Family Therapy uses stories, fables, and myths. One experience that corresponds to stories in many ways is the dream. It is a very personal story whose meaning and significance are not immediately apparent, but hidden in symbols. While the dream represents an individual mythology, stories and sayings are collective mythologies. They, too, contain symbols and hidden information. They originate not in the individual preconscious working through of conflicts, but in the tradition of the society that produces them. The goal of therapeutic stories is not so much moral teaching, but the imaginary association with a model situation. Stories thus fulfill a number of functions.

MIRROR FUNCTION

The multitude of images in stories bring their contents closer to the individual and makes it easier for him to identify with them. The listener can structure the assertions in the stories in ways that correspond to his own psychic structures at that particular moment. In the stories he sees himself as if he were looking in a mirror.

MODEL FUNCTION

Stories present conflict situations and set forth possible solutions or point to the consequences of particular attempts to solve them.

MEDIATOR FUNCTION

A direct attack on misunderstandings, resistance, and defense mechanisms usually triggers a responsive defense that is equally intense. In the psychotherapeutic situation, the confrontation between therapist and patient is eased by the insertion of stories as a medium between the two "fronts." It is a sign of respect for the patient, acknowledges his narcissistic desires (cf. R. Battegay, 1977, 1979), and offers him a shield that enables him at least provisionally to deal with his defense mechanisms.

STORAGE FUNCTION

Because of their imagery and the emotional resonance they can evoke, stories are easily remembered. They are not only present in the therapeutic situation, but also in the patient's everyday life. As similar situations call them to mind, the need exists to think about the questions raised by the story.

STORIES AS TRANSCULTURAL TRANSMITTERS

As bearers of tradition, stories become representatives of cultures. They reflect the game rules, concepts, and behavioral norms at work in the culture. These contents in the stories provide the members of a society with strength and reassurance. They set forth solutions that are acceptable in a particular cultural circle. Stories from other cultures, on the other hand, bring information about the game rules valid in that culture and enable the listener to expand his repertoire of concepts and to see them in more relative terms.

STORIES AS AIDS TO REGRESSION

The medium that is addressed by stories is intuition and fantasy. Within our achievement-oriented society, the return to fantasy is interpreted as a regression, a backsliding to earlier stages of development. In the therapeutic framework, stories make it possible for the adult to cast off the armor of acquired behavior he has learned—at least on an experimental basis—and to again adopt earlier, pleasure-oriented behaviors and attitudes.

STORIES AS COUNTERCONCEPTS

By using a story, a therapist does not present a prescribed theory, but offers the patient a counterconcept that he can accept or reject. One identifies in part with the alien view and sees just what parts of it are acceptable for his particular situation, how it can give him a better picture of reality, and what cannot be applied to his specific case.

In the psychotherapeutic situation, counterconcepts are offered as *prescriptions* (Watzlawick et al. 1969; Selvini et al., 1977). The patient is given the task of grappling with the counterconcept. This can mean: read a story, think about it, talk about it, or write down your understanding of it. The therapist can prescribe this expressly or—without pointing it out in particular—let its challenging nature lead the patient to practice the counterconcept on his own. The form one selects for the counterconcept is likewise dependent on the circumstances: stories that present the information with a lot of redundancies and poetic imagery; the "moral" of the story, where the informative concept is summarized briefly; a saying or proverb that is particularly apt; a "formless" counterconcept that arises directly as the answer to what the patient has offered.

The majority of our stories go beyond pure description and contain a conversion experience similar to what one knows from optical illusions: without costing the listener or reader a lot of trouble, he accomplishes a change of perspective that comes as a surprise and provokes an "ah-hah" experience. But there is something else that goes along with the change of perspective: Familiar situations are seen from a new point of view, which gives them a different character. Sometimes this change of perspective by itself is the solution to the problem.

I have compiled a number of Middle Eastern stories that, if used at the right time, can be beneficial to the course of the therapy (Peseschkian, 1979). In so doing, we consciously go back to elements of a prescientific folk therapy and try to intergrate them into the scientific concept of Positive Family Therapy.

SELF-DISCOVERY

As with many other things, we have *learned* our relationship to stories, fables, and fairy tales. We have learned to love them, to be indifferent toward them, or to reject them. There are some questions that can help us better understand the background of our attitudes toward stories:

1. Who read or told stories to you (father, mother, siblings, grandparents, aunt, kindergarten teacher, et cetera)?
2. Can you remember situations where stories were told to you? How did you feel?
3. What do you think of fairy tales and stories?
4. Which story, tale, or fairy tale comes to mind right now?
5. Which sayings and concepts have the greatest meaning for you?

Some people develop a great fondness for the metaphoric language of stories, but some have a deeply rooted mistrust and aversion to them. But sometimes this is actually more a dislike for their religious, philosophical, and family connections than for the stories themselves. In the case of my book *The Merchant and the Parrot* (1982), which deals with stories and their application in psychotherapy, I found that some readers were concerned because they could not apply the stories although they had a keen sense for stories. Almost equally often, I found that in the families they grew up in, a lot of value had been placed on "politeness" while telling jokes and witty stories had been taboo. This shows that it is good to inquire about such matters.

Part VIII.

Concepts and Their Effects in Positive Family Therapy

An Everyday Example from Medical Practice

A patient comes to the office. He looks exhausted, acts restless and nervous, and huddles on the examination table like a lump of bad luck. Only with great difficulty is he able to describe his complaints. He has sharp pains in his left arm; his heart pounds rapidly as if ready to burst out of his body. At night when he is in bed, his heart hurts as if he were having a heart attack. He feels sick to his stomach and is plagued by the fear that he will have a heart attack at any minute. The doctor listens to all of this patiently and formulates in his mind the proper diagnosis. His own experience forces him to acknowledge that it could be a case of functional heart trouble. After a thorough physical examination, the doctor arrived at a conclusion: functional heart disease. As an experienced doctor, he began to ask "When did the pains grow worse? Do you feel under a lot of pressure at home or at work?" The patient nodded. The doctor had touched on a sore point. Now the patient spewed it out like a waterfall: "I take over assignments for colleagues, have new projects going at work, feel insecure, get more and more work dumped on me, and can't say no. My wife doesn't understand what's going on; she thinks I'm a failure. I can't even really help my son. He'll probably flunk this year."

The doctor listens to these complaints and prescribes sedatives and medication to stabilize the man's circulatory system. As he leads him to the door, he shakes the patient's hand, gives him a friendly pat on the shoulder, and offers a bit of advice: "Don't let yourself get so worked up over things, take it a little slower, and, most of all, do something about all that stress."

Outside, at the doorway, the patient mutters, "But how?"

There seems to be a dilemma in customary psychotherapeutic practice in that, on the one hand, the initial interview, which has basically a diagnostic function, is confused with therapy itself. The diagnostic process leads to the idea that therapy has already taken place: "You, the patient, know what matters."

On the other hand, there is a game of psychotherapeutic blindman's buff. Out of fear of being biased, one dispenses with giving a diagnostic judgment, which, at any rate, is never final in terms of a clinical diagnosis. Simply because the patient has come to therapy, one believes he has to run him through the therapeutic mill without first explaining thoroughly whether therapy is called for, which kind of therapy should be used, and what therapeutic goal can be set, at least provisionally. These decisions, not the mere labeling of cases, are the main tasks of the diagnosis.

Differential analysis uses a multileveled plan of treatment that can be regarded as the guideline for differentiation analytical psychotherapy. It is understood primarily as interaction.

The following cases illustrate how concepts affect the family situation and how the tools of Positive Family Therapy can be used.

1. Frigidity: The Ability to Say No with One's Body

One example of the positive process is the way we deal with the problem of frigidity. More than anyone else, the gynecologist deals with this phenomenon. It is an instance that gives rise to many problems. Often there is no detectable physical cause for it, and connections with hormonal disorders are more the exception than the rule. Nor can genetic disorders be accepted as the cause in most cases. This leaves only psychosomatic considerations—and here the practicing gynecologist is often rather helpless. One cause for the difficulty is the illness designation of frigidity itself. It assumes that the woman carries this frigidity around as a health defect, just like a growth in the uterus. What we mean by the positive process can be illustrated by the following case.

A thirty-two–year–old married woman, Ursula F., came to therapy with her husband. When asked what she was suffering from, her husband immediately answered for her, "My wife has sexual problems. She's frigid." He said this with a strength of conviction that stunned me. He used the term "frigid" like a firm diagnosis:

> *Therapist: "How do you know that?"*
> *Mr. F.: "Our family doctor said so."*
> *Therapist: "You know this only from your doctor?"*
> *Mr. F. (obviously embarrassed): "I had already felt from time to time that my wife was rejecting me sexually. But I first knew it was a case of frigidity when my wife went to the gynecologist and our family doctor read the findings to us."*

He accepted the diagnoses that had been presented by the specialist. It seems interesting that the diagnosis of frigidity is simply a description of the quality of the sex life. It takes the side of the man, who perceives his wife as cold and negative. This experience, moreover, is to him akin to a far-reaching narcissistic illness. Mrs. F. was hurt by his aggressively proclaimed statement. In contrast to her husband, she began to describe her problem by telling me that she felt depressed and thought her relationship with her husband was in trouble. She had gone to a gynecologist because of a vaginal discharge and had also told him that sexually she felt nothing but disgust and resistance.

It seemed to me that the woman had taken on the "blame" for the problems the couple was having. Her husband made all sorts of efforts, but despite it all, she just couldn't join in. The increased efforts to have a satisfying sex life produced just the opposite—namely, deep feelings of failure. Her frigidity was viewed as an organic inferiority; their efforts to deal with it had brought them to a therapeutic dead end.

But there exists another way of understanding this disorder. In this case, frigidity is a sexual defense and represents the attempt to avoid sexual and marital confrontations simply by withdrawing. It is more than sexual coldness. It is *the ability to say no with your body.*

When I suggested this counterconcept to the couple, they were both speechless. I feared they wouldn't know where to start with this interpretation, but the wife then began to discuss the problem from her perspective: "A long time ago, I gave up saying no to my husband. He never has time for me, you see. He's married to his job and comes home when he feels like it. He's been doing that for eight years." She said her feelings seems to be aimed most at defense. When she thought about having to endure sex, she tensed up. Her last satisfying sexual experience had been seven or eight years ago.

The positive reinterpretation made it possible to see the problem at a new level and to approach it from new aspects, such as the husband's job activities (industry/achievement), his lack of time, his unreliability and tardiness, the wife's concept of justice, as she no longer wanted to put up with these shortcomings on the part of her husband, and her difficulty in expressing her discomfort with and asserting herself against her husband (politeness/honesty). The symptom of frigidity is thus not simply an abnormal characteristic of the woman. Rather, it is an expression of the disturbed emotions and communication in the relationship.

By not repeating the illness concept, we acquired new ways to deal with the problem in accordance with family therapy.

In the course of the five-phase therapy, which included fifteen sessions over a period of ten months, we were able to achieve considerable improvement in the wife's health, but even

more important was the noticeable change in the family's communication structure. The prerequisite for this, however, was our leaving the well-worn paths of conventional diagnosis and establishing new perspectives with the patients so that existing problems could be viewed in a new light.

2. What Do Stomach Troubles Have to Do with Frugality?

Food to a man is like oil to a lamp: if it has much, it shines, if too little, it is quenched; yet a lamp is sooner extinguished by too much oil than by too little.

—Oriental wisdom

Hartmut O.: "My pains have gotten worse in the last six months. I suddenly get stomachaches after I eat. Even if I'm slightly upset, I get a full feeling in my stomach. And on top of that, I start sweating when anything unexpected happens. Because of these problems, I don't feel I can accomplish much. And I'm also afraid the condition will get worse. Already I feel I can't do as much as I'd like. . . . The trouble started shortly after one department was moved from the company headquarters to a remote location. At the same time, I got word that my former boss wanted to come to the home office. I had had a lot of trouble with him when we worked together at the branch office. This news was therefore a great shock for me."

—Excerpt from initial interview

Mr. O. presented his problem as a conflict at work. Based on his descriptions, I would have almost been tempted to interpret his problem as excessive professional demands and authority conflicts. His fussy manners gave me the impression that he had a compulsive personality structure. But his pains and his description of himself did not make his suggestion as to how his stomach problems had developed plausible. X rays had already led to a diagnosis of gastric ulcers. Compared to this organic symptom, the psychic symptoms remained in the background. The patient spoke about feeling upset and how this always went right to his stomach. He also mentioned being afraid the pains would get worse. He stubbornly had nothing to say about the contents of his anxieties. These fears, by the way, were not the result but the conditions of his physical problems. With regard to his sweating problem, however, Mr. O. was able to report that the periods of excessive perspiring came on him like attacks and were perhaps the equivalent of suppressed anxieties. It wasn't at all hard for him to describe the way he dealt with conflict: "I react to conflict with my body and with my imagination. In that respect, I'm just like my wife. Whenever she gets upset, she gets a headache."

This was the first time he mentioned his wife, and he presented her in such a way that she almost had as much right to be a patient as he. He hinted that in addition to his problems at work, there were also troubles in the family. Mr. O had developed quite a good career as an engineer, and, to use his own terms, "now he was somebody." He enjoyed this feeling, even if he felt somewhat pressured by the academic engineers under him and by his boss. His wife, so he said, had given up her job as a buyer and now lived for her family—that is, her husband and sixteen-year-old son. Neither parent seemed to be very sociable. Half ironic, half convinced, Mr. O commented, "Cozy home, but happy alone."

When asked what concepts were important for him, he said without further ado, "At our house, the motto was 'What comes to the table gets eaten.' On this point my parents and, even more so, my aunt wouldn't give an inch. And achievement got a lot of emphasis in our family, too. What I am I owe to the fact that I was always told to strive for the top. And thrift was another important thing."

It was precisely the theme "frugality" that Mr. O seized upon while working through the DAI. He seemed quite fascinated by it. As an assignment, Mr. O. was asked to describe the conflict situations in which his stomach pains occurred and to pay particular attention to his relationship to the concept of frugality. At the next session, the following dialogue took place:

> *Therapist: "You wanted to observe your experiences with your stomach problems and with the theme of frugality. What did you discover?"*
>
> *Mr. O.: "Well, I thought about the whole problem and wrote down the questions. And just as I had written down the questions, I realized that I'm actually very stingy. I was so upset and shocked by this realization that I tore up what I had written and don't have the documents I had promised I'd bring for you. But I can tell you what I wrote down. It occurred to me that I am the only one in the family who rolls up the tube of toothpaste so the last bit can be squeezed out of the tube. My wife and son just let it lying there any old way, and that bothers me.*

"And marmalade is another thing. When you spoon it out of the jar, a bit always sticks to the rim. Well, when the marmalade gets low. I take a spoon to push it from the rim back into the jar.

"Another example is my driving. I never do it when it's risky—such as in the mountains—but otherwise I put the car into neutral when I go downhill. I mean, if I can maintain the same speed going downhill, I put it in neutral. This saves gas.

"The next thing I should mention is eating in restaurants, which I bascially don't like to do because I really hate to spend money on things I can get cheaper at home and of the same quality, because my wife is an excellent cook. But again I must admit that this is just a disguise for my greed. When we eat out, I always make my selection quickly and order first so that I can set certain limits on the prices. But my son, who could care less about such things, orders what appeals to him, and it's usually something expensive. It makes me mad that he ignores my hints, and then I get a pressure in my stomach, and this is already the start of the problems that lead to a bad stomachache after the meal.

"Whenever I have a business lunch or even eat socially with other people, I wait to see who offers to pay or I try to suggest that we each pay our own. As soon as a decision is made, and we either pay separately or together, the pressure on my stomach goes away.

"I thought of another thing: I like to putter around the house and have even built a few things by myself. Whenever possible, I try to straighten out bent nails I've pulled out of a shelf or something so I can reuse them. It never occurs to me to throw away screws or used or bent nails. I keep all sorts of things like that. I even have a box where I keep things I can't use immediately. I know I'll put them to good use someday."

Therapist: "What about clothes and things at home?"

Mr. O.: "I wear my things a long time. I already told you I have a jacket I've been wearing for fifteen years. Not the trousers, of course, but the jacket. I've even worn it here once. A brown jacket is always in style. Over the years, pants change more than jackets do. And actually, when I go to work I change clothes and put on a uniform so my good clothes don't get dirty. I'm sure this is also why I have back problems. My job requires that I pick up stones weighing as much as forty pounds and then hit them with a hammer. It would be easier for me if I propped them up a bit against my stomach. But I don't do that. I hold them out with my hands so that I don't get my clothes dirty. That way they don't have to be washed so often, which is another way to save money."

Therapist: "You have taken a close look at yourself. But what about that motto, 'What comes to the table gets eaten'?"

Mr. O.: "Oh, yeah. When I didn't want to eat because I didn't like it, I had to stand in the corner until I was ready to eat all my soup. At that time, we lived with an aunt in East Prussia. She had a rooming house for girls who came from the countryside to attend school. I had to stand in the corner in front of all those girls. I was probably nine or ten then. I think this is also why I really felt embarrassed for someone, like my boss, for instance, when he somehow said something ridiculous after a lecture. This public display, even if it didn't involve me, caused me to break out into a sweat. Even today, when so-and-so asks a dumb question in the middle of a discussion, I just boil inside."

Therapist: "Do you see any connection with your illness?"

Mr. O.: "You had told me the story of someone who got fat because he had lost his provider. [The therapist had briefly mentioned the case of "John" as an example of physical and mental connections.] I blame my overweight, my potbelly, on the fact that when I'm invited to dinner, even on business, I eat everything. Again, this is part of my greed. After all, I don't need to eat everything, because basically I'm satisfied after a moderate portion. But since it has to be paid for anyway, I feel obliged to eat it all. That's a point that also follows the same pattern."

This interview with Hartmut O. clearly shows the demands that his family had made regarding thrift and nourishment. To be sure, his comments dealt with familiar behavior, but they were so new to him that he was again and again surprised to see the connections that he could make with the theme of thrift. They were play forms of an emphasized concept of frugality and had come to dominate many areas of his life. His attitude toward his body was just as influenced by his frugality as was his family interaction, his contact with other people, and his situation at work. His thrift, which led him to shortchange the other areas, was directed toward a still indefinite future. Mr. O. was tormented by the idea that the future might bring changes that could cause him to lose his job and be unemployed in his old age. As a result of these ideas, he felt he had to rely on what he could accumulate through his own efforts.

After we thoroughly discussed the theme of thrift (the stage of observation) and Mr. O. had gotten insight into the connection between thrift and emotional tension, we investigated the autobiographical background to these concepts (the stage of inventory). The means by which we explored this area were the four model dimensions. Mr. O. was an only child. He felt more drawn to his father, a very industrious and thrifty man, than his mother. Mr. O. said he had always respected his father, but with his mother there had often been conflicts. She was, so he said, a fanatic when it came to neatness ("just like my wife)": "If I tyrannize my family with my frugality, my wife does it with her sense of orderliness."

His parents, who were still alive, had an unusually stable marriage. He had never been abel to identify problems that could have destroyed the marriage. And for him, family and marriage were equally important: "If I need a sense of security from somewhere, I can get it only from my family. As the breadwinner, I am responsible for taking care of external matters." His parents had little contact with other people, but the father was somewhat more sociable than the mother. The father had seen to it that the family, despite all the difficulties, did not lack what it needed. The mother, on the other hand, had paid more attention to religious matters: "My father was too materialistic for that. He always said, 'I'd rather be a sparrow with my savings account passbook in my hand than a bird of paradise strutting about on the roof.' "

At the third stage, the stage of situational encouragement, we dealt primarily with the positive aspects of thrift. Mr. O. was quite taken aback by this, because he had been expecting criticism. In particular, we talked about how thrift provided safety and security and how important these feelings were for Mr. O. We also discussed the fact that thrift meant self-reliance and independence for him, especially independence from paternal authority, a force that he identified with very closely. By discussing these things, Mr. O. became more aware of the guilt feelings that had continued to lie in the background.

The verbalization stage was characterized by my posing counterconcepts to the concepts that Mr. O. presented. This took place through transcultural examples: "In the Middle East, thrift takes on a different form—even from the point of view of safety and security. One uses money for social purposes, thereby strengthening one's social contacts and creating the right to be taken care of by other people if circumstances make it necessary."

This way of dealing with the problem of security was a new perspective for Mr. O., as he said himself. Other counterconcepts that helped bring about a change of perspective were contained in stories such as the story about "expensive thrift." In the story, a man has to take on a number of burdens in order to save money, but in the end he has to pay out money anyway (Peseschkian, 1977, p. 197; 1979, p. 105).

At the stage of verbalization, Mr. O. began to set up a family group. Up till then, his treatment had been individual therapy, with his parental family and his own family treated in an "imaginary" way. But now the family was directly involved. Themes that became acute in the course of the first session with the family group were still those of Mr. O.'s frugality as well as his wife's pronounced need for neatness.

After the ninth session, the stage of goal expansion became the focus of the treatment. In this sense, it wasn't treatment anymore, but a kind of controlled self-help. The family group had already become a solid institution. In goal expansion, Mr. O., in conjunction with his family, tried to activate the areas that had been previously neglected. At the same time, however, this meant that his concept of thrift lost its severity. He spent money for tennis equipment, signed up for tennis lessons, and thus fulfilled a wish that he had had for a long time, but had suppressed because he thought it was frivolous. On business trips, he began ordering better food, stayed at better hotels, and no longer tried to save money on petty expenses. He seemed more capable of enjoying himself and less encumbered by his compulsive thrift.

The amazing thing was the social skills he developed. Along with his wife, he built up a circle of friends, and it was not at all hard for him to buy them a meal from time to time, or to give them gifts.

When we said good-bye after the twelfth session, he said, "I still like to feel financially secure. But now I also get a real sense of security from my wife and my new friends."

3. My Parents Raised Me Wrong

One may tell the truth—even to one's father.
—Oriental wisdom

For many people, child psychotherapy has this meaning: The therapist takes on the parents' responsibility for raising the child and tries to correct existing behavioral and experiential characteristics. One begins to consider the possibility that not just the child alone, but also the family game rules influence the origin and course of the disorder. And this leads to the realization that the family itself should be treated. To put it bluntly, psychotherapy for the child means psychotherapy for the parents.

This is easily understood if we keep our eyes on how the parents, consciously or unconsciously, exert an influence on their children. The child thus plays the role of the symptom carrier; he may be the black sheep, the scapegoat. His symptom is an expression of the communication disorder within the family. Providing isolated therapy for the child alone is dangerous for two reasons: For one thing, the psychotherapeutic situation, where there is no punishment, begins to compete with the parental home, and the contrast between the two simply strengthens the unsatisfying situation the child finds himself in. And second, child therapy, in a pure form, means that the conditions that favored the development of the child's behavioral disorder will continue, creating new conflicts for the child.

Psychotherapy for the child, like family therapy, is thus directed primarily at the parents, who then acquire therapeutic tasks. The relational persons (father, mother) themselves adopt the emotional portion of the therapy with the child. As a rule, the question is not how more love and attention can be given to the child, but which capabilities are favored or suppressed through which form of attention. This sharpens the competition between the relational persons (the parents) and the psychotherapist. The latter here takes on a function that is quite similar to the processes of a fermenting agent. He introduces processes of self-help and controls the course of the events that have been begun. If the parents are not willing to cooperate, it is often better to forego an isolated treatment for the patient than to add fire to an already heated atmosphere by bringing in a psychotherapist.

In the long run, reeducation (psychotherapy) as a corrective measure cannot be limited to the relationship among child, parents, and therapist, but must also take into consideration other educational institutions (school) and the informal "teachers" in the social environment. These may be friendly or hostile to children. In a certain way, kindergarten and grade-school teachers are substitute parents. Because of the society's demands for achievement, these teachers expect the development of individual actual capabilities. In so doing, they can evoke or reduce conflicts and, to a certain extent, carry out some therapeutic functions.

A mother and her twelve-year-old son came to therapy because she "couldn't deal with him anymore." She reported, "I don't know what's gotten into the boy. The way he's been developing the last few years, I'm afraid he could become a criminal. At night he steals large sums of money from our cash box and denies everything afterwards. We got a lot of complaints from school that he was picking fights with older boys. Since my son thinks a lot of his father, we tried to use a trick to make him come to his senses. My husband took some time off and went to a spa, and we told the boy that his dad had had a heart attack because of all the trouble with him and that he had had to go off to get some rest. I noticed that the boy felt guilty, but the results didn't last for long. We had some sessions with an educational counselor and with a psychologist, but after a year of treatment nothing had changed. . . ."

The son gave his version: "When I take money, I'm so upset I can't sleep right. I really hate school. When I sit down to do homework in the evening, I get very restless."

Conspicuous aspects of the boy's behavior were related to school, to problems arising in connection with school, and to occasional thievery.

The Differentiation Analytical Inventory (DAI) revealed the following areas as being conflict-laden:

> *Punctuality:* "Mark doesn't come right home from school. All I can do is keep supper warm for him and hope that he's not gotten himself into trouble again. . . ." "The boy used to have to wait for me a lot. I had promised to help him with his homework. But usually something came up at work, and Mark waited for me for

hours because I couldn't get in touch with him. . . ."

Orderliness: "We used to have a cleaning lady. But now she doesn't come on a regular basis. But my son would never hit upon the idea that he should at least keep his room cleaned up."

Honesty: "That's the main problem for us. We don't know who he gets this stealing from. If he keeps it up, we just won't be able to trust him anymore. And I am haunted by the fear that sometime he might steal something big and be labeled as a thief. . . ."

Industry (School): "In school he does the least work possible. He's always got other things on his mind. His teacher told him that if he keeps it up, he'll never graduate. . . ."

Thrift: "He doesn't know how to handle money. When he steals money, he uses it to buy toys for his friends and gets nothing out of it for himself. . . . We've told him he can get money from us any time he needs it, he doesn't need to steal. But he steals on the sly anyway. . . . He's never gotten an allowance. Why should he? After all, he can always come to us when he needs something. . . ."

Contact: "He hardly has any friends. He's close with only two school chums, and they aren't the right company for him. He rarely brings kids to the house. Usually we invite business acquaintances. Mark has protested, 'Always the old people.' "

The boy's dishonesty was related to his need for contact with his peers and for recognition from them. For Mark, money was a way to get attention from his classmates as well as from his parents. But he had never really learned how to associate with them. His ability to trust his parents, especially his mother, had already suffered before his parents' trust was called into question by his thievery: Mark had had to wait for his mother for hours and thus discovered that school really couldn't be so important after all, since his mother didn't seem all that concerned about it. The parents' guilt feelings led them to transfer Mark to another school when problems began to emerge. The result was a series of school changes within a short time. Here again the boy seemed to get a particular message: "You don't need to worry about doing well. We'll jump right in when things go wrong."

At first, the boy's therapy was unsuccessful. It seemed as if the therapist was supposed to become an ally of the boy against the parents, who seemed to be to blame for everything: "My parents simply raised me wrong. How can I help that?" The therapist became more and more a confidant for the boy. He became a person whom the boy could tell things he wouldn't say to his parents. I showed him that he had an array of qualities and couldn't be as bad as his environment and finally he himself claimed he was.

But the main weight of the treatment lay with the parents. The mother was not included in the therapy, but received "therapeutic tasks" anyway. She was able to consult with me at certain times. Within twenty-five sessions, the treatment was terminated.

4. Adiposity

Fill a third of your stomach with food a third with drink and leave a third of your stomach empty; then, should anger seize you, there will be room for its rage.

—Oriental wisdom

When there are psychosomatic disorders, it is good to examine the concepts that are connected to the conflictual behavior and experience. Concepts are the central point of a conflict, not just in the case of dramatic psychic alterations, but also precisely in those cases that seem to be the result of bad habits.

An example of this is John F., a forty-four–year–old technician who is five-ten and weighs 275 pounds. As in most cases of overweight, there was no evidence of a metabolism disorder. On the one hand, John suffered a great deal because of his weight. For about six months, he had been treated for diabetes and also showed visible signs of high blood pressure. But, on the other hand, he seemed to have fatalistically accepted his overweight as fate. At the persistent urgings of his family doctor, he had started therapy. The doctor had worked with him for a long time, but had found that diets, health spas, and fasting at fat farms had been worthless. John gave the impression that he felt utterly superfluous in therapy. He looked with interest at the furnishings in the room and clearly appeared to be ignoring me. The start of the treatment was very difficult. The patient hardly said a word except for some general comments about his family, his career path, and about how he had gotten used to being laughed at because of his weight. He claimed he had no more complexes about it.

When we got to the subject of John's concepts, the following dialogue took place:

Therapist: "What did your parents put more value on? On food, on doing well in school, on being together as a family? Or did everyone simply go his own way??

John: "They were always concerned about school. But it was particularly important that we eat together. My mother was an excellent cook. When I was worried or upset about something, she was espcially good to me and made my favorite dishes." [*John stops his description as if it were painful for him to talk about his family's eating habits.*]

Therpist: "What motto seemed to determine things at your house?"

John: "In our house, there was no question about that. The motto was 'Food keeps body and soul together.' I can clearly remember that whenever I didn't want to eat, I was told, 'What comes to the table gets eaten.' . . . If I couldn't finish my lunch, I got it warmed up again for supper. When I didn't want to eat, the word was 'There's nothing else.' Every piece of bread that I started to eat I had to polish off. [*John laughs pensively.*] *And we were really a terror when we ate in a restaurant. The food we consumed there! We had our own motto: 'Rather make yourself sick than leave something for the owner.' I still heed that rule today. At my company's picnics, there's never food left; I eat it all. My buddies make fun of me: 'Rather get a belly from eating than a bad back from working.' "(John smiles contentedly; beads of sweat appear on his red forehead.)*

The patient's concepts regarding food and nourishment extended back into his childhood. Here we came upon an experience that had great significance for John. When he was nine years old, his father died. It was wartime and soon the postwar era came. Food was scarce and John's mother complained constantly, "What will we do now that our provider is dead?"

The father's role crystallized in his function as breadwinner, and this conception fo the father role remained in John's mind. Food thus took on a symbolic character. It became for John a symbol of the trust and security that he associated with his father. The idea of the provider being dead and the unconscious conclusion that he himself would starve led John to assure himself again and again that there was still enough to eat. This is why he ate as much as he could and enjoyed with every bit a strong feeling of security. In doing so, he fit right in with the family's traditions regarding food. Even today, as he told us, his grandmother still saw to it that he ate enough. When he returned home in the morning after working the night shift, he couldn't go to bed until he'd eaten a meal. His grandmother would even wake him up if she discovered he hadn't eaten.

This collection of concepts was more than merely a justificational ideology for John. He regarded them as assertions that greatly determined his self-image. He could identify with them because he had grown up with them and because they represented the epitome of attention, security, and achievment. They were the center in his system through which most of his motives, goals, and wishes passed. As long as the concepts had unlimited meaning for him, all attempts to lose weight permanently were futile. John's preferred area for dealing with conflict was his relationship to his body. He was a gourmet cook and a gourmand, an epicure and a glutton. With so much emphasis placed on the body, there was a corresponding deficit in the area of social contact. Aside from his mother and grandmother and a few colleagues at work, John had hardly anyone he could consider a friend. He had an excuse that he proclaimed in a convincing manner: "If I work overtime every week, how can I have time for friends and company?" Very subtly, almost as an afterthought, he added, "What would I do with house guests? First of all they cost money, and, second, I'd have to provide food, which makes me fat." John was indeed a model of industry and thrift. He frequently volunteered for overtime and also saw to it that he got put on shifts that paid better. His very apparent industriousness was thus rooted in his thrift. This need, however, was again related to a concept that we have already become familiar with: he had to have a big-enough financial cushion that would guarantee that he always had enough to eat. In this connection, John thought of stories about POWs who, even years after their release, could not fall asleep at night unless they had a bit of bread under their pillows. They had simply not been able to overcome the memories of the starvation they had suffered years before.

Despite the vividness with which John was able to report on his eating and his gorgings, contact with other people seemed unable to draw him out of his reclusiveness. He was strongly affected by comments to the effect that human contact is part of man's nature and that he needed and had the capacity for contact as much as he did the need to eat. But these comments did not lead him to talk about it. His onesidedness led me to think of the story of the shared commandments. This story tells of a mullah who heeded only the first part of the command "Eat and drink, but in moderation." The mullah let other people heed the second part, but disregarded it himself. I told the story to John. He used it as a reason to talk about how he would like to have a girlfriend but had not yet had a serious or lasting relationship because of his physical appearance. But here again his frugality helped him make a virtue out of a vice: "A wife would cost me a pretty penny." But in contrast to how he had spoken earlier, John said this with an ironic gleam in his eye and was clearly less serious about what he was saying. As a counterconcept, and to expand his concepts, I told John about the importance of contact in the Middle East, about how extensive the family relationships can be, and how contact can be used to enhance one's sense of security and self-esteem. Thinking in terms of differentiation, John saw the connection between his thriftiness and his eating and the substitute function they had—initially for his deceased father and then for social contacts with other people.

Up until then, the focus was on the stage of observation and inventory. Through this, John gained access to his problem. At the stage of situational encouragement and verbalization, John was able to try out new points of view, at first experimentally and reluctantly, but later with curiosity and eventually with energy and thoroughness. This was the situation when we terminated the treatment. The fifth stage, goal expansion, had already been laid out, of course, but by then I could not and did not need to help John any more.

The actual therapeutic treatment lasted fifteen sessions. During the last seven sessions, John followed a diet at home.

A half-year after the termination of therapy, John came to my office again. He gave a fresh and lively impression and exuded the same calm and assuredness as earlier, but was otherwise hardly recognizable. He was sixty pounds lighter, was now more interested in sports, and was planning an extensive trip during which he would participate in sports activities. His blood pressure was now normal, and he no longer needed treatment for diabetes. His weight loss had relieved his metabolism of fats so greatly that the insulin production from the salivary glands in his stomach was now adequate for his needs. But this had not come about simply by a single act of will, but through changes in his attitude and the expansion of his concepts.

5. A Heart Neurosis

If I say something and am considered bad because of it, that's still better than if I say nothing and am considered as stupid as a donkey.

—Oriental wisdom

A thirty-six–year–old Iranian, Behzad, was manager of a large travel agency. He had been living in Germany for several years and was married to a German. When he came to me for psychotherapy, he already had an odyssey of medical treatments behind him. For five years, he had been complaining about circulatory problems, which expressed themselves as problems in keeping balance, dizziness, and headaches, as well as heart pains on the left side, irregular heartbeat, depression, and anxiety. With these symptoms, he had already been able to baffle a number of doctors in Iran and in West Germany. But no one had found a physical cause for the problems. Treatment with medication for heart ailments did not alleviate the problem; on the contrary, it simply made the heart more and more the center of attention. The occurrence of disorders became more and more noticeable. When it became apparent that psychic disorders were the source of the problem, psychological drugs were used. First Valium and Librium, then antidepressants were used. But this treatment likewise failed to produce the desired results.

As the initial interview, the patient seemed to be a sensitive, receptive, extremely polite, and considerate person. He kept apologizing for being a problem for me. But even more clearly did he express his dependency wishes: "You are my last hope." As an only child, Behzad had grown up almost exclusively with women who, as he told it, had fussed over him in a loving and demonstrative manner. These women included his mother, his grandmother, two unmarried aunts, and some cousins, who all took turns spoiling Behzad. Very early on, he developed into a charmer who knew exactly how to get the love and attention of his "women." Even when it was thrown up at him that he wasn't a "good" tough fellow, the attention of the women in his family seemed more important to him than fighting to assert himself. Even later on, he preferred having women around him rather than men, he said. At home, the system including many women functioned without complication.

But when he arrived in Germany five years ago and married a German woman, his problems began. But his wife was not the actual partner in the conflict. The DAI showed that there were few significant conflict areas between the two. The problem actually was with the patient's "old women." Just as in earlier times, they now still wanted him in their decision processes, to help them with their purchases, big and little problems, travel plans, and such. But now he felt completely helpless in the face of the many demands they made on him. His problem was that he could never say no. During our initial interview the following dialogue took place:

> *Behzad: "I can't stand it anymore. I've got an awful headache."*
> *Therapist: "You are troubled by a lot of things. That's what's causing the headache."*
> *Behzad: "That's for sure. They just won't leave me alone."*
> *Therapist: "Who, exactly, is not leaving you alone?"*
> *Behzad: "My mother, my aunts, my grandmother. They all always want something from me. I don't have any time at all for myself and my family."*

It seemed that the headache was Behzad's symbol for the many expectations and concerns that his relatives piled on him. At the end of the sessions, I returned again to Behzad's problem with politeness, which seemed to be the center of his conflict situation. It seemed connected to emotional reserve, his desire for security and maternal recognition, on the one hand, and for self-assertion, independence, and integrity on the other:

> *Therapist: "Have you ever tried to tell them you can't do everything?"*
> *Behzad: "That's completely out of the question. They've done so much for me. I can't hurt them. That would be mean and unthinkable."*

Behzad had reacted vehemently. It seemed like I had touched a neuralgic point that was loaded with guilt feelings, anxiety, suppressed aggression, and a distorted sense of gratitude and indebtedness. As an assignment for the next session, I gave him a Persian proverb: "If I say something and am considered bad because of it, that's still better than if I say nothing and am considered as stupid as a donkey."

At the next session, Behzad immediately took up this theme: "I find this proverb marvelous. It really fits my situation. How often have I been dumb as a donkey and haven't said what was bothering me. While driving I've been singing this proverb to different tunes that come to mind. My wife has been wondering what's gotten into me, particularly because I have to laugh about this sometimes and she doesn't know why I am laughing. Somehow, I feel very relieved about things." But despite this enthusiasm, Behzad had second thoughts: "If I say what's on my mind, the others will be mad at me, and I'm not sure I can endure that."

These thoughts indicated that Behzad was harboring quite a bit of aggression. Just as water can build up behind a dam, a number of aggressions had collected behind his friendly and communicative facade of politeness. And he was afraid the dam would break. He mistrusted these suppressed forces so much that he didn't want to even allow them the kind of release that would have taken place through an open and honest mode of behavior on his part. As an assignment for the next session, I told him the following proverb: "The person who makes a lot of noise and spectacle should not be feared, but the one who pulls in his head and remains silent."

Behzad thought about this assignment for a long time. "I've been thinking about something that I just can't put out of my mind. If this is really true, then it follows that by swallowing everything, I have much more rage, anger, and aggression that if I would express my opinion on this and that."

With these comments, Behzad was trying a new perspective, initially on the cognitive level. This became the turning point for the therapy. In subsequent sessions, I gave him other assignments, such as "A Reason to Be Thankful (see page 00)."

It was apparent that Behzad was gaining insight into his conflicts and the factors that were troubling him. Through change in perspective, he also learned other answers to his conflicts; in particular, he learned to distinguish between his own wishes and those of other people. The treatment lasted twelve sessions and spanned eight months. His circulatory problems and heart ailment, which we virtually ignored in our therapeutic talks, diminished. Significant depression no longer occurred.

6. "What Will People Say?"

You may regret your silence once, but you will regret your words often.

—Oriental wisdom

A thirty-two–year–old woman had requested a meeting with me. She was dressed very stylishly and made an elegant impression on me. But her appearance was marred by her somewhat nervous gestures and her restlessness. She explained her wish for psychological treatment this way: She said she just hadn't been able to manage things for a while. "I feel depressed, empty, and burnt out. Nothing interests me anymore, and everything bores me terribly. I don't have a real relationship with my husband anymore. I'm totally indifferent to sex. Lately, I've even been thinking it might be better if I divorced him." In fact, the patient gave an impression of hopelessness and seemed to be expecting to be told that that was indeed her problem and that nothing could be done to help her.

We set up an appointment and decided that the next time she should bring her husband along. Despite her doubts that it would be possible to get him to come to therapy, the two arrived at the set time. But now there was an astonishing change in roles. It wasn't the patient who complained about her problems. Rather, the husband presented himself as the one who was suffering, as the one who needed the therapist's support: "Between me and my wife are two walls and four steel-plated barricades. I simply can't get through to her. I'm suffering terribly from this." The wife turned aside, as if she weren't interested in his complaint, and adjusted her makeup. Her husband continued. "That already started soon after we got married. That was five years ago."

"That's been a problem in both my private life and at work," he continued. "I'm irritable, impatient, and get caught making mistakes I used to never make before."

I then asked them to tell me about the situations that led to their fights. In the ensuing conversation, I used the model of the four areas for dealing with conflict and the Differentiation Analytical Inventory (DAI).

The wife used my question as a starting point to describe with great vehemence a series of situations. She spoke so emotionally that her husband hardly came through with his weak protests: "Since we've been married," the wife said, "my husband has looked at me as little more than a cleaning lady. I used to have a good job at a bank. I could go out with people on my own. But today I'm only there to vacuum the carpets, wash dishes, and straighten out the throw rugs." She stood up, walked over to the rug, and actually began to smooth out the fringes. Her husband protested, "Don't act so silly." But she didn't let that bother her. She said, "I feel like a slave. My husband is the pasha. He travels around the world on his business trips, learns to know thousands of people, and I sit here and play Cinderella."

Her husband interrupted her. "Don't carry on as if it's all my fault. I have to get up at six in the morning. And when do you get up? I make my own breakfast. And when I call you at eleven, your're usually still in bed."

These accusations seemed too much for the woman. With anger that she could not suppress, she snapped back, "That's it. That's precisely it. If I wake up early, I know the whole day is meaningless and that I can't motivate myself with housework. The thought is simply too much for me."

At this point, I suggested that maybe a cleaning lady could help. Their reaction was astonishing solidarity from both of them. Both the husband and the wife protested against this idea: "That costs too much, it wouldn't work, and what would our in-laws say? They wouldn't like the idea at all."

I then asked where the in-laws lived and how often they came to visit.

"My parents live about 250 miles from here," replied the man, "and they come here two or three times a year."

Somehow there seemed to be a discrepancy between the in-laws' actual influence and the respect the couple seemed to bestow on them.

What that all meant became more clear in the succeeding conversation. We had been talking about cleanliness and neatness and had determined that both partners put extreme importance on these behavioral areas.

Then the wife told of the following experience: "A colleague of my husband came to visit, and I had gotten everything ready. Walking around the room, he ran his fingers along the moulding, looked disgustedly at the dust, and then blew it away from his fingers like this.

[She demonstrates.] And he said, 'As a housewife, you certainly aren't breaking your back.' This experience hurt me deeply. And my in-laws do the same thing. I always get the feeling they are trying to show how incompetent I am as a housewife."

At this point her husband jumped in: "This is exactly why I insist that everything be neat. I don't want both of us to be blamed in front of my parents. When things get chaotic around here, I have to ask myself, 'What would people say?' " Here the husband had hit on the key conflict in his marriage. This "What will people say" was for him an attempt to prove to them that he could handle everything with his wife, in spite of everything. With his colleagues, his perfectionism required him to be "spotless" both at home and on the job. The same concept was operating for his wife, although from a different point of view.

It occurred to me that the question "What will people say?" enveloped the marriage like a gloomy phantom. This fear seemed to be present at all times. What was missing was the realization of whether or not the anxiety was justified. For this reason, I took over the concept of the family in the positive process. I reformulated it in only one point: "Find out for yourselves what people really say." I assigned the couple the task of behaving in such a way as they considered proper and asked them to observe the actual reactions of other people, to write them down, and to report on them at the next session. The focus was on the real reactions, but not on how the couple thought the others would react.

I tried to help the couple understand the sense of this procedure by telling them two stories. The first story "A Reason to be Thankful," demonstrates that honesty often helps the partner more than politeness does. Politeness, of course, can protect the partner, but often misleads him. The second story, "The Difficulty of Doing the Right Thing For Everyone, (page 00), which the couple recalled again and again, dealt with the difficulty of being all things to all people (Peseschkian, 1982). It shows that regardless of what one does, one's critics will find something wrong with it. Even if one does nothing because of fear of doing something wrong, he is not spared some criticism. Now and then it is unavoidable that we step on someone's toes. Here we find the concept that one must learn to live with the risk of occasionally losing the friendship of another person.

At the next session, the two spoke almost exclusively about the experiences with other people. They had tried out various strategies and techniques to find out what the othesrs would say. They provoked discussions, challenged their neighbors and colleagues to express their opinions, and even got their in-laws, who had come for a visit, to say what was on their mind.

At the third session, the husband commented with astonishment, "It's really not as bad as I had expected. In my mind I've always been worse than now, now that I have heard what other people think of me. They don't have such a bad opinion. I have suffered more from my politeness than I now do from the people's honesty."

His wife added, "The funny thing is that the others criticize me once in a while, but the criticism doesn't bother me anymore."

In the course of the therapy, which amounted to eight sessions over a period of four months, the two partners tried to differentiate their relationship to each other and to the in-laws and to work out the permanent areas of conflict. For them as for me, it was surprising that problems that seemed to be vicious circles lost their force as soon as a counterconcept was presented.

7. Literary Concepts: Who Is Your Favorite Author?

Those who do not help others need doctors to help them.
—Oriental wisdom

The literature on family and psychotherapy would give the impression that ultimately concrete personal relationships determine the milieu for a person's upbringing. But alongside these personal relationships we are connected in a network of concepts that are associated with individual persons, of course, but go far beyond them. There are concepts of imaginary people, and these concepts branch into one's own concept system and either strengthen it or call it into question.

For this reason literature is of special importance. It is the medium by which a society gathers a considerable part of its concepts and ideologies. It thus fills a representational role: literature reflects what the reader himself thinks and feels. Literary concepts thus become an object of psychotherapy. They gives clues to the cognitive structures and the conflict-laden concepts of the individual. He does not find himself solely in the concrete family group, the peer group, et cetera, but also, by means of his concepts, in an imaginary group that is linked by a philosophically transmitted "sense of we." Insight into this collective mythology is provided by the questions of which collective mythologies one adheres to and with which world views, philosophers, religious leaders, ideologies, writers, or scientific approaches one at least partically identifies. This question is of therapeutic significance, because the preferred concept program is not unchangeable. Rather, it needs constant reaffirmation, if one leans towards experiences that support the concept and relies on other concepts that call the other ones into questions.

In psychotherapeutic practice, we actually observe a conspicuous relationship between relational problems and the personality structures and a preference for individual writers. I found, for example, that a number of patients undergoing a serious identity crisis selected Nietzsche and Hermann Hesse as their favorite writers. Included in this group were patients with generation conflicts, alcoholics, schizophrenics, and people suffering from depression. These concepts accompany a person throughout his life or seem typical of the crises of growing up. Interwoven with his life story, they become characteristic features that help us sketch a "psychogram."

When we establish such a connection for an individual patient or a group of people, the preference for one writer or for a particular type of literary concept is not an absolute diagnostic clue. The real purpose for isolating literary concepts is not primarily a diagnostic investigation, but an aid for better understanding.

A fifty-six–year–old engineer came to my office because of a retirement process. He appeared to be very depressed. He sat stiffly in his armchair and hardly showed any facial expression as he described his problems in short, choppy sentences. He seemed to wear a wrinkled mask that reflected depression and pessimism. He was not very talkative. The little he said was simply information in catchwords: "Heart attack two years ago, difficulty with concentrating. My doctor says I should retire." Aside from these complaints and a brief summary of his life, there was not much to discover. He was, as one calls such people in psychotherapy, an unproductive patient, one who mainly uses language for silence. Since I didn't get much more through direct questions, I tried to determine how he reacted to conflict. I was particularly struck by his affective repudiation of social contact:

Patient: "When I come home, I want my peace and quiet."

Therapist: "Do you do much with your wife and kids?"

Patient: "I can't, and I wouldn't want to either."

Therapist: "Let's assume you'll live another twenty years. Do you want to continue living so isolated and lonely?"

Patient: "I've lived like this for fifty-six years, so I can do it for another twenty years. You can't do anything about your fate. You are what you are. You can't simply do an about-face."

Therapist: "What do you do instead of that?"

Patient: "I read books."

Therapist: "What kind, if I may ask? Who's your favorite author?"

Patient: "Schopenhauer!"

Therapist: "What do you particularly remember about him?"

Patient: "Well, there's a saying of his that means a lot to me: 'Fate shuffles the deck, and we play.'

Therapist: "What does this saying say to you?"

Patient: "That it is all a matter of fate and that we can't do much about it. I've always been a quiet, withdrawn person, and you can't change that!"

Therapist: "I know a similar saying from the Persian poet Saadi: 'Even though everyone is fated to die, don't put your head in the mouth of the lion!'"

Patient (after a period of silence): "I never heard this version before." (He again becomes silent and, deep in thought, is obviously interested).

Therapist: "Whos is your favorite writer besides Schopenhauer?"

Patient: "Gottfried Benn. He wasn't successful in dealing with his fate either. . . . He became melancholy. . . . But he regained his equilibrium through his writing."

Therapist: "What is it that you like about him so much?"

Patient: "For one thing, that one experiences his sorrows. And then there's a sentence of his that means a lot to me: 'Silence is more than truth.'"

Therapist: "How has this saying affected your life?"

Patient: "I can be happy by myself, too. Why should I quarrel with my wife? Everybody should know for himself what he can do and what he should leave alone."

Therapist: "What other author comes to mind?"

Patient: "Well, there's Goethe. In his conversations with Eckermann, he said, 'Regardless of what happens, life is good.' But I have trouble with this sentence. It's exactly the opposite of what I think."

I noticed that the patient spoke much more freely and openly when he wasn't the goal of the investigation, but when he could talk about his literary interests and the concepts contained in them. It was easier for him to present Schopenhauer's or Benn's ideas than to describe his own being. In the patient's statements, he outlined a number of conflicts that could have been worked through in ensuing psychotherapy. The openness that he exhibited was especially surprising in view of the background of his generally closed and withdrawn personality, his reserve, and his silence about matters concerning his inner life. At this discussion, it was not yet determined whether there would actually be psychotherapy. But the patient seemed very open: "My work is really the focal point of my life, and I don't know if it's such a good idea for me to retire already."

When he left, he asked me to write down Saadi's saying for him, "because I'd like to think about it some more." This form of self-depiction, of course, does not provide an exact description of biographical data, but does present important qualities about one's perceptions and aspects that, on the one hand, come from a definite psychic development, but, on the other hand, introduce this development (in the form of the parents' basic concepts) and intensify them (as one's own attitudinal and behavioral concepts). The literary tradition is filled with such concepts, which arose from a particular situation and now serve as a model, as an aid to understanding, and as an outline for the interpretation of analogous life situations. Perhaps this relationship is one reason why literature and art speak to us so powerfully. They reflect situations and problems that are also important for us and reveal connections that we can use for our own guidelines. Literary concepts offer an almost unending reservoir of counterconcepts and concepts that can expand one's horizons. They provide alternatives to the interpretational scenarios from which conflicts originate. In this sense, we can draw on the sayings of other writers and poets or on the sayings of the same poet in order to look at a literary concept in a new light.

It is precisely this case depiction that shows that a cultural system of relationships contains well-formulated concepts that can help a person learn to understand himself. Of course, which concepts are chosen depends on the developmental conditions in question. And part of these conditions are the family backgrounds embedded in the social processes.

Part IX.

Family Tradition and Identity

1. Traditional Neurosis

THE DIFFICULTY OF DOING THE RIGHT THING FOR EVERYONE

In the heat of the day, a father went through the dusty streets of Keshan with his son and a donkey. The father sat on the donkey, and the boy led it. "The poor kid," said a passerby. "His short little legs try to keep up with the donkey. How can that man sit there so lazily on the donkey when he sees that the boy is running himself ragged?" The father took this comment to heart, climbed down from the donkey at the next corner, and let the boy climb up. But it wasn't long before a passerby again raised his voice and said, "What a disgrace! The little brat sits up there like a sultan while his poor old father runs alongside." This remark hurt the boy very much, and he asked his father to sit behind him on the donkey. "Have you ever seen anything like that?" griped a veiled woman. "Such cruelty to animals. The poor donkey's back is sagging, and that old good-for-nothing and his son lounge around as if it were a divan—the poor creature!" The targets of this criticism looked at each other and, without saying a word, climbed down from the donkey. But they had barely gone a few steps when a stranger poked fun at them by saying, "Thank heavens I'm not that stupid. Why do you two walk your donkey when he doesn't do you any good, when he doesn't even carry one of you?" The father shoved a handful of straw into the donkey's mouth and laid his hand on his son's shoulder. "Regardless of what we do," he said, "there's someone who disagrees with it. I think we have to know for ourselves what we think is right."

". . . But since I have just said that our ancestors should serve as our model, the first exception to this must be that we don't imitate their mistakes." This text from the first of the *Three Books of the Duties,* by the Roman politican and writer Cicero, can be the motto for the following section.

The family presents itself in the therapeutic situation and exposes its typical forms of interaction. We find their sources in the personal experiences and the common history of the group entity "family." Like roots, they go beyond the concrete family situation back into the history of past generations. In order to understand a family's situation, we must know the situation that existed in the parents' family of origin. At this point, we are dealing with the grandparents and could go back into the family history even further and trace the tradition of symptoms, conflicts, and strategies for solving them.

Two things happen in this process: For one thing, one becomes aware that peculiarities have grown in a historical way and are thus not absolute, but have relative meaning. Many things that are looked at superficially and then labelled as "endogenous," "inherent," and "linked to the character" have their origins in family transmissions. They remain hidden from those who fail to inquire about them. Second, one gains more understanding of the mechanisms by which these family traditions are transmitted. They are "game rules of the second rank" and determine how obligatory the family concepts really are and what adherence they require: "Changing one's mind is a form of betrayal or a sign of a weak character"; "What do I care what I said yesterday?"; and "I have to rethink my position again and again."

The question of guilt, in the sense of personal responsibility, appears in a different light. Against the background of family delegations, one can understand behavioral forms that would otherwise simply be regarded as deviant or morally questionable.

In the form of concepts that intensify or change in the course of the individual life, in the interaction of family and social groups, and in the transmission from one generation to the next, the word *heritage* derives its particular meaning. Even when the rigid forms of transmission are opened up and a unilinear tradition is replaced by a pluralistic one, origin is an essential factor of one's identify. Shakespeare wrote in King Lear: "A person who scorns his ancestry can never again be firmly rooted in himself." The dissolution of old tribal relationships and obligations to the clan have limited the sociological significance of the family of origin, of course.

In the sense of invisible loyalties (Boszormenyi-Nagy and Spark, 1973) and the family and cultural concepts that also mark the relationships of the groups to each other, the "tribe" still exerts considerable influence on a person's identity.

2. Hanging onto Concepts or Changing Them

Don't limit a child to your own learning, for he was born in another time.

—Rabbinic saying

The word *elevate* is understood in terms of Hegelian dialectics as both preserving and changing at the same time. Here we find connecting points with conflicts. Preserved concepts strengthen the family loyalty; changed concepts go hand in hand with a process of detachment or restructuring of the family. The relationship between two generations becomes the welding joint of tradition. There are various kinds of loyalty and thus a loyalty conflict. It can become an insurmountable problem if one has to choose between the father's suggestion and the mother's, for example. Such a decision is accompanied by direct and immediate consequences: "My daughter has become the same kind of slob as my wife. When I see her running around in her rags, I can't help being angry," says a forty-three–year–old civil servant who grew up in a family of government officials and married a musician. In a similar way, family loyalties can become conflicts when the partners cling to their concepts while no one is willing to relinquish his responsibilities to his family origin, even if such a change would enable the partnership to forge a new identity: "My husband is just as pedantic as his father. He expects me to be just as fussy. I'm proud of the fact that my parents raised me in an easygoing way and that warmth and social interaction were more important to them than good grades in school," says the wife of the government official as she describes the problem as she sees it.

A further way of reacting is to rebel against family traditions. This repudiation can take place in various ways. It can result in coquetry with regard to parental authority: "When I moved away from home for the first time, the first thing I did was take a school friend to my apartment and sleep with him. I didn't particularly like him, but I did it because I wanted to do something that my parents, those stiff old pillars of virtue, would have forbidden," says the eighteen-year-old daughter of white-collar parents who forbade sex, partly for religious reasons.

The protest against traditional concepts can also be demonstrated by declaring one's cessation of loyalty to the family and developing ties to other social systems. A common example of this is the intertwining of political and religious convictions with the generation problem. For example, one fights paternal concepts and tries to establish his own concepts and to affirm them in the struggle against family and community authority. This way of looking at things, of course, disregards the contents of the conflicts but does describe individual important features of the psychology of participation and solidarity. Here again the process can develop over several generations so that the repudiation of paternal ideology still stands within the family tradition. A twenty-two–year–old student, after long and bitter confrontations, finally distanced himself from his family, whom he labeled as bourgeois, materialistic, and too much a part of the establishment. His father was an entrepreneur who had started his own business and felt completely misunderstood by his son. But this conflict repeated the confrontations that the father had had with his father-in-law. The latter was a laborer and socialist and viewed his son-in-law's ambitions with reserve. Soon there was a conflict that spanned three grenerations, for the grandfather and the son took sides in a family struggle against the father. The problem, which had political aspects to it, became linked to a conflict based on psychological and family problems. Psychotherapy and family therapy deal primarily with the latter. By becoming more aware of the personal and family aspects, the political demands and the political discussion can also be shaped in a more differentiated way. The father one clashes with is a problem; the problem of social justice is not the same. This distinction makes it possible to have a constructive conflict. The conflict is then no longer mere confrontation and hate that degenerates into speechlessness. It becomes an interpersonal problem that can be solved or can at least be clarified to some extent.

At this point, examining the family tradition can help clarify matters. The son perceives himself simply as split off and isolated from his family. When the grandfather supports him in the therapeutic family group, he comes to understand himself within the political and philosophical traditions of the family.

3. The Undecided Generation Conflict

The Golden Mean is to love this world, to do good in life, and to aspire to the world to come.

—Saadia Gaon

When two people start a family, they bring along their own set of concepts. They work out specific arrangements. Either they are in a position to develop a living relationship with each other, thereby establishing a lot of trust by developing mutually held concepts that represent a compromise, or their individual loyalties to their respective families can determine the scenario (Boszormenyi-Nagy and Spark, Sperling, and Sperling, 1976). One or both partners clings to his and/or her family's concepts and finds only a few areas of common ground where the relationship can gain a foothold. A child growing up in a such a situation will have difficulties. If he identifies with the mother's concepts, he repudiates the father. If he adopts the father's ideas, he opposed the mother. Regardless of whose values the child accepts, this decision is always accompanied by guilt, by the feeling of having hurt the parents. And with this guilt there is a need to correct the wrong as quickly as possible. This occurs again when one goes beyond the family and establishes ties to other people and groups. The parental arrangement will be repeated. But here, instead of a having to make a choice, the individual finds a seat between two chairs.

Concepts can continue from generation to generation. Often they perpetuate themselves over several generations, causing problems when social and family situations undergo basic changes and the old program no longer has an answer for this new situation.

WHEN CONCEPTS BECOME RELATIONSHIP TRAPS

Clinging to traditions transmitted by the family, even if they are long-held traditions, can lead to a dead end. Traditional concepts have their own ambivalence, which is not always visible to the individual, and this ambivalence can cause a lot of suffering.

The resolve with which one upholds definite family concepts is, paradoxically, not always rewarded. Often, in fact, there is a kind of punishment, which in particular cases is represented by expulsion from the traditional family community.

4. Till Death Do You Part

If things are not as you like, like them as they are.
—Oriental wisdom

A forty-three–year–old woman, Hilda L., had gotten a divorce after twenty-one years of marriage. This resulted in such great turmoil for her that she saw no other way out than to attempt suicide. After she had recovered physically, she came to me for psychotherapy. The impression she made was that of someone homely and plain. A bit on the plump side, she seemed to me like a little gray mouse. Her clothes were neat, but looked homemade. In a soft voice she told me about her problems. From time to time she interrupted her descriptions to sob and cry, "I can't sleep at all anymore. I'm really through. Since I got my divorce I don't even feel human anymore. I keep thinking about how this all happened. But I don't have any explanation about how this all happened. But I just can't figure it out. I'm so depressed and sad. Three weeks ago, it was so bad I really wanted to die. I took some sleeping pills and wanted to just end it all. . . ." The problems began about two months after her divorce. What had happened? The husband of the patient had entered into an extramarital relationship. Mrs. L. didn't think she could put up with that. For her, the injury her husband had inflicted on her through his infidelity was simply too great. In this idea she was supported by her religious and family concepts. For her, fidelity was the basis for trust between partners and was the most essential element in marriage. Going hand in hand with her depressed, clinging personality structure was the concept of faithfulness till death. The model her parents presented strengthened her in this, for in their narrow family circle they shielded her from external influences and silently disapproved of any attempts to break out of it. The moral commands of her church likewise advocated fidelity and declared infidelity to be a sin. Given this background, she found her husband's adultery to be unbearable. Here the first relationship trap had already slammed shut. The patient had paid scant attention to her physical appearance. Although she kept her home in perfect shape, she neglected herself. As she had learned at home, she stayed in her apartment except to go shopping from time to time or to visit relatives. She didn't like company except for birthdays and holidays. As far as sex was concerned, she was also quite conservative: "Why should I get all dolled up and act like a tramp? That's not my style." She behaved like the dutiful daughter who diligently tried to live up to all of her parents' wishes. For her husband, who enjoyed people, this was a signal to look for sexual satisfaction and social contact elsewhere, even in places that his fantasy led him to. For the behavior that his wife indirectly drove him to he was punished with her withdrawal and the divorce. All his pleading for forgiveness and his promises to never do it again fell on deaf ears. In her eyes, his wayward steps had discredited him forever. He was someone she could no longer trust. But at the same time, her constant emphasis on fidelity backfired on her. Instead of being rewarded for her steady adherence to the principle of faithfulness, she was criticized for getting a divorce—not because she had been unfaithful, but because she had stood up for fidelity to the bitter end. At the same time, her family turned against her. She was particularly hurt by the fact that one of her aunts, a nun who had taught her the importance of fidelity and the uncompromising nature of faithfulness, reproached her. Mrs. L's parents made it known to her that, as a divorced woman, she was no longer welcome in the family. As they saw it, she should have not been so egotistical in proclaiming how right she was. After all, they reminded her, the command was "till death do you part." So the second relationship trap slammed shut. Suddenly the patient was standing all alone and had lost the support of the very family whose beliefs had forced her to risk a separation from her husband. The results were disappointment, fears of being abandoned, and the feeling that she had been treated unfairly and dishonestly. She also felt severely depressed, at least until her attempted suicide.

The therapeutic process was geared toward making the patient aware of the existing concepts and somehow reeducating her to the possibility of looking at alternative concepts that could perhaps help her resolve her problem.

5. The Wrong Way

Let us be like the lines that lead to the center of a circle, uniting there, and not like parallel lines, which never join.

—Oriental wisdom

In our society, *education* is usually synonymous with "education for achievement." This is why we come upon a typical relationship trap with astonishing frequency.

A successful architect had married a woman seven years younger than himself. He wanted to offer her everything. In order to have the house of his dreams, he worked like a machine. There was hardly any free time for him. Overtime was the general rule, and when he came home tired, he told his wife about the successes and progress he had made. In return, so he said, he could expect love, attention, and security. At first, his wife accepted these things from him. She lived like a wife and mother in her golden cage, a cage that she could not leave. Her desire to take up her old work as a secretary or at least to help her husband at the office was rejected by him as if it were an insult: "As if I couldn't take care of you!" Their seemingly idyllic life burst like a bubble when the child-wife met an artist who—as her husband said—was still wet behind the ears and couldn't do much but put on a big act. The fact that this man gave the wife something that the husband couldn't did not become apparent to the husband until much later. Those things that the artist could give were vision and time. The husband, on the other hand, had learned that you win warmth, love, and attention through your achievements and your industriousness. This concept led him to expend himself on business activities and to overlook the fact that a partnership can be based on entirely different criteria. The well-intentioned upbringing he got from his parents turned out to be a relationship trap with its own delayed ignition system. It was a trap that he set for himself in his choice of a spouse and in the way he shaped his marriage.

Regardless of which field of psychotherapy, self-help, or education one deals with, it is important to be alert to these relationship traps. The actual capabilities, the model dimensions, and the four forms for dealing with conflict represent particular detection devices for uncovering these traps.

6. Delegated Concepts

From happiness to sorrow takes a moment; from sorrow to happiness takes years.

—Oriental wisdom

Concepts are contained avowedly and unavowedly as game rules in interpersonal relationships. To some extent, one formulates his concepts clearly and succinctly and says, "Orderliness is half of life." But, on the other hand, one lives them without being aware of them. One straightens a picture hanging a bit crookedly on the wall, picks up every little dust ball off the floor, and feels comfortable only when the house is as tidy as he wants it to be. Concepts are passed on between the generations in a similar two-fold way: By saying what kind of order one wants and by living that order, punishing the child or mate for alleged sloppiness and tending to the same area until the other person identifies with it or runs away from it: "We don't invite our mother-in-law here anymore. She always has to show us that my wife is not the ideal housewife. She never passes up an opportunity to show how careless my wife is."

The microtraumas, the so-called little things, are not coincidental. They represent definite concepts in the social environment. Since the parents are the ones who influence a person from early childhood on, they are also the ones who can prepare the first neuralgic points for microtraumas. Without making the concepts obvious, they transmit them "drop by drop." These ideas can then coalesce in the child's experiences and develop into concepts. The child notices how he should behave and how he shouldn't; he notices what's good and what's bad and combines these individual concepts with the image he has of himself:

"My mother has to come home on time. Otherwise I get scared. I have to come home on time; otherwise my mother starts to worry, and then I get punished. If I'm not punctual, the others get mad at me and reject me."

This developmental chain was one we found in the case of a thirty-five–year–old compulsively structured patient, who in turn victimized his own family by making punctuality the first commandment and tardiness an unpardonable sin.

In a similar way, we are nursed with concepts, so to speak, from infancy on, and our concepts are then re-formed according to the particular features of our situation.

But the development of the concept can be uncovered not only for the life story of an individual, but also over the course of several generations. When we inquire into the causes of a concept, we can examine a cross section. What shape does the concept take in a person, his parents, and social subsystems and within the socially approved behavioral code?

We can also make a longitudinal study as to how a concept has changed and been shaped through a person's life and even over the course of generations. This way of looking at it is like the search for the historical roots of an individual and the group with which he feels some common connections. Here one can understand the terms "rootedness" and "lack of roots." A person is uprooted when entrance to the history of his individual and group identity is cut off. To draw his family tree, a person generally only tries to document his biological heritage. Sometimes this is for the purpose of growing generation-long membership in a particular social class, such as the nobility, or in a particular racial group (Aryan). Some find it a special sign of prestige if they can point to a famous person among their ancestors. But, as Plutarch once said, "It's nice to be from a good family, but accomplishment is only becoming to one's ancestors."

In recent times, some social groups have thought about their collective history and origins in order to define their historical and social situation. At the same time, this makes it evident that one is part of a developmental chain that is stamped by society to some degree.

In Positive Family Therapy, the *concept family tree* helps make the developmental conditions more apparent. A family tree or family chart shows the ancestors of a couple. In a similar way, a concept family tree contains the source of development undergone by a concept as it went from the parents to their children, grandchildren, and so on. This process is of particular interest for studying the development of a concept but is not practical in the therapeutic situation. So we use this technique for the table of ancestors: We start with the patient or patient family and try to recall the concepts that were valid with their ancestors. Despite the differences between an ancestry table and a family tree, we have adopted the meaningful term "concept family tree," even though it is not completely correct.

The actual capabilities and the forms for dealing with conflict are a guideline for the journey into the past. As far back as the family transmission extends, we inquire about which concepts a member of the family represents and how they have changed during his life. We are able to pose these questions to members of the child generation, the parental generation, the generation of grandparents, and, indirectly, even to members of generations preceding them.

7. The Old Prohibition

Why did God create Adam alone? In order to teach us that whoever destroys a single life is as guilty as though he had destroyed the entire world and that whoever saves one life earns as much merit as though he had saved the entire world.

—Talmud

The members of a family became aware of the significance of their uncritical adoption of ideas on religion. An actual conflict had developed when a twenty-four–year–old man wanted to marry a Catholic woman. Although his parents and siblings claimed that they no longer adhered to the traditions of their Protestant faith and that they thought church was a lot of nonsense, the religious difference suddenly became a problem. It could have been decided to limit the therapy discussion to questions of how to solve this problem, but I went a step further and, together with the family, tried to follow the development of the religious concepts.

Except for the "rebel," they were all in agreement on one point: namely, that you couldn't trust a Catholic very far. As far as they could remember, there had never been a marriage with a Catholic in their family. Developing the concept family tree became an exciting type of detective work, going back to the great-grandparents. A long-forgotten family document came to light, indicating Huguenot ancestry on both sides of the family. The great-grandfather on the paternal side was one of several Protestant pastors mentioned in the document. He had been known as an ardent fighter for the Protestant faith. The grandfather was a businessman, considered by all to be a good Christian, who regularly attended church.

But the parents had loosened their connections to the church considerably. They had seen to it that their children were confirmed, of course, but otherwise, like Ibsen, they considered religion to be a lie. But even so, their dislike for Catholics, an inheritance from those forefathers who had been exiled by the Catholics, had persisted and now, in connection with the son's problem, had become the material for an acute conflict. After the family tradition had been explained and understood and the parents had gained insight into the unconscious processes by which the concept had been delegated, it was much easier for them to go into their current problem, which was no longer veiled by the concept of hatred for the Catholics.

The guidelines for the concept family tree were the actual capabilities for faith/religion, contact, justice, and honesty. Many wishes, demands, and reactions that seem unfounded at the moment are concepts can be traced back in the family tree, thereby acquiring some particular meaning. But this meaning is frequently found several generations back and is revealed to a certain extent only much later.

8. Dangerous Tea

People treat each other in a friendly fashion—when times are good.

—Oriental wisdom

I observed similar concept traditions in a different cultural connection when I looked at Iranians who had lived in Europe for more than a decade. Just as fossils emerge out of the ground, so there appeared concepts that surprised them themselves. An Iranian engineer on a visit to Germany told me, "When I found out that you are a Baha'i, I just got a knot in my stomach. I actually felt sick. I didn't think I could finish the tea I was drinking. I almost had to throw up."

I was startled by this powerful emotional reaction. My visitor was a confirmed Shiite. We had often had dealings with each other, so that he trusted me enough to be willing to pursue with me the causes for his reaction.

My guest told how he had often quarreled with his father, who apathetically prayed the suras of the Koran without understanding a word of it. He himself couldn't accept that, and when he attended the Koran school he delved into the religious texts. But this was not sufficient reason for his strong aversion to me, an aversion that caused him to feel physically ill. The key to this secret was found in the engineer's grandfather. In his youth, the grandfather had been very involved in religious questions and had come into contact with some Baha'i. But he soon withdrew from this contact. Some of his friends had become Baha'i, a change of belief that he regarded with scepticism and some anxiety. He based his reactions on an explanation that was common in Iran at that time. The mullahs said that the Baha'i tea contained a powder that made one easily impressionable and no longer able to defend his own beliefs. The engineer had heard this from his father and grandfather when he was a child. As a result, he had avoided the company of Baha'i and, particularly, their mysterious tea whenever possible.

Here the family chronicle again touches an acute symptoms. One day, before the engineer had a sudden attack of nausea, we had tea together and talked about religious questions and the problems of political developments in Iran. Right then he remembered the moment he had happened to find out that I was a Baha'i. His subsequent nausea was an attempt to get rid of the danger in a symbolic way. Unconsciously, in the sense of an "organ language," he tried to get rid of the "dangerous tea." The roots of his reaction were guilt feelings with regard to his own religious concepts and those transmitted to him through his family. This was confirmed in our discussions. We talked about the fact that, despite his religious convictions, he had some doubts about his faith and his unexpected meeting with a Baha'i was a double threat to him.

These connections really caught his interest. We discussed this theme for a long time. A few weeks later, he sent me a letter and said he had had similar problems with other colleagues and that their fanaticism and prejudices troubled him greatly.

9. Can One Hurt Other People?

A man who never leaves his home is like a man who spends his life in prison.

—Oriental wisdom

The transmitted concepts can accompany a person's concept family tree for several generations. Some of them have their origins in crucial experiences of family members, who then pass their experiences on to their followers. But other concepts are based primarily on philosophical and religious utterances. Within the family, they take on such weight that family life is regulated according to them. As suprafamily concepts, they go beyond the family itself and determine the family members' relationships with people of the same belief and conviction as well as with people who represent other ways of thought.

Here it is found that the in-group and out-group relationship remains surprisingly stable over the course of several generations. The same holds true for the structures of the family, which are transmitted as being specific for the culture or the group. The constancy and durability of these structures and relationships stem from the concepts. The following case is an example of a transmitted concept that suddenly takes on special meaning in the life of the individual.

A medical student was suffering from recurring attacks of circulatory distress. In the course of his psychotherapeutic treatment, he spoke of severe conflicts of conscience. It was impossible, he said, for him to use the scalpel or the hypodermic needles on people. We then searched for the concepts behind his fears. Socially, there is an expressed command against harming other people. For the patient, this command was underscored by the religious traditions in his family. He was of the Jewish faith, which forbids a strict follower to touch his face—God's image—with sharp metal. In accordance with this view, strict Jews do not shave at all or do it with a wooden razor. The patient wanted to become a doctor. It is peculiar to the medical profession that its practitioners are permitted and required to do injury to the human body. Surgery, injections, punctures, et cetera are everyday practices in medicine. In conflict with the religious and social idea that the body must not be harmed, there is the requirement of the medical profession that inflicting pain is necessary to keep a human alive.

But this description of the conflict does not explain it entirely. After all, there are plenty of doctors who are not troubled by this conflict. We therefore investigate what a physical injury means in the patient's family and what importance it gives to the body, pain, and physical integrity. We discovered that the family relationships were very polite and that aggression was inhibited. Conflicts were expressed intellectually, particularly by the dominating mother. Reason was the most frequent means of overcoming a conflict. Physical force, even the patient's fighting while playing with other children, was viewed as ugly and unworthy. All these components were mirrored in a specific way in the patient's personality, needs, and anxieties.

Against this background, which was differentiated and analysed more thoroughly during the treatment, the patient's anxiety about using needles or scalpels became understandable: as an expression of his desire to avoid threat to his self-esteem ("only a barbarian would physically hurt another person") and a threat to the economy of the personality ("When I have the scalpel in my hand, I could hurt my father or mother or my siblings"), as representative of his fear of losing love ("If you put yourself outside the law and are disobedient, you no longer belong to us"), and as representative of his fear of going against religious commandments.

This example shows how clinging to family concepts and role assignments can lead to difficulties when a person suddenly considers ways of acting that were either not present in the original concept system or were even forbidden by it.

10. The Redeemer

We each have the kind of children we deserve.
—Nachman of Bratslav

Problematic attitudes and tasks can grow out of a family and continue over several generations until finally one person takes over the task of breaking the family out of its rut. Anxiety, compulsive rituals, and dependencies that gave the family its mark are conquered through the active intervention of the family member. The following case is a typical example. A young man takes on the task of freeing his family from hypochrondriacal fears that had persisted for several generations.

There were already pronounced signs of hypochrondria in the second generation. The grandparents were fortunate if they could take care of their children and grandchildren. There was always a half-fearful, half-joyous expectation of the worst illnesses. This was repeated in the parents' generation. The father denied his own feelings and fears, but was always threatened by heart attacks. But the threat diminished when his wife became sick. She suffered periodically from depression and a constantly recurring fear of cancer, which she feared would strike any of a number of organs. The son, who was in intense competition with his father, followed the family tradition in his own way. Since childhood, there had been only one profession that interested him: medicine.

Despite a flirtation with psychotherapy, in medical school and later on in his practice, he concentrated on themes that are appropriate for getting rid of his anxiety: he specialized in forms of incurable cancer.

11. The Concept Family Tree

If you don't teach the ox to plow when he's young, it will be difficult to teach him when he is grown.

—Oriental wisdom

A family of three came to my practice. The nineteen-year-old son was introduced as the patient. He seemed withdrawn and negative. The parents summed it up this way: "Our son is the black sheep of the family and must be gotten back on the right track."

His symptoms were impressive. Classical psychiatry would have called him an uncontrollable psychopath. He drank a lot, got himself into drunken brawls, and, so his parents said, hung around with bad companion to whom he was almost a slave and had also been dabbling with hashish and other drugs. He didn't have a job. Even though he had done average work in school, he had quit shortly before graduating.

The young man confirmed what they said and mentioned that he had trouble concentrating. He simply couldn't live up to the expectations his parents had for him: "They're just shitty bourgeois. The only thing that matters with them is 'work and earn and see to it that you have things better than the next guy.' " In fact, the father, who was forty-eight, reported that he had an incredible amount of work to do as a corporate lawyer and was afraid that all the pressures would lead to a heart attack. The mother tried to smooth things out, saying again and again, "We only want the best for you." This sentence became a key statement.

On his own, the father began telling about his parents and his childhood: "I'm the oldest of three kids and have always upheld the family order. That has served me well. I have made a success of myself, and I'm proud of that. But I'm not proud of my son. He has been a disappointment. On the other hand, we haven't had a bit of trouble with his older brother. He's more like the family."

I asked the father to talk more about his childhood and his own parents and grandparents. His father had had a small company in the man's hometown, employing several people, and his mother had been a very industrious person. She had grown up in a poor family, but had taught her son a lot about ambition and persistence: "There was a good sense of order in our family. We knew exactly where we stood. Our motto was 'Nothing comes easy.' I've accomplished more in my life than ten people like my son could ever do."

The man's grandfather had been a self-made man who had built up a nice business out of a small shop. But it seemed hard for the father to continue talking about his ancestry. Finally he recalled that his great-grandparents had moved from the country into the city and that things hadn't gone well for them at first. He ended his family chronicle by talking only about the developments in the generations on his father's side: "In our family, things always got better. We've all made something of ourselves. You can imagine how it hurts to see that our son has turned out so different. What could I have done with him?"

The son sat there and listened with keen interest.

I asked the mother to tell about her family. She had come from a lower class family and been raised to "make something of herself." Her parents made great sacrifices so that she could finish school, and she even went to college and studied German and art history for a few semesters before she met her husband and got married. The surroundings she grew up in and still represented were summarized in the concept "What will people say?" She felt pressured to achieve something so as to bring honor to her family: "My mother was so proud when I went to high school. She told everyone how well I was doing in school."

The woman's mother had also taught her how to be a good homemaker, and at this she was a real expert. Her kitchen absolutely sparkled, and her living room looked like it belonged in a magazine. I asked the mother where her mother had learned to place so much emphasis on housekeeping. Her reply came rather hesitatingly: "My grandmother was a servant girl. My mother learned a lot from her. We kept house just like the fine folks."

The actual capabilities that one notices in this family tradition were orderliness, frugality, and politeness, with also some weight placed on achievement and prestige. They had to at least keep up the image of social respectability and the impression that they felt they belonged to a higher social class.

We were able to develop a concept family tree containing the concepts transmitted through the family. This family tree can be seen in counterpoint with the social and historical conditions that accompanied the change in the concepts.

The family tree was developed as the family members tried to recall the important concepts of their ancestors as they had heard of them in family stories. In the family tree, one can clearly see a tendency for advancement on both the paternal and maternal sides. This tendency goes hand in hand with the lower–middle-class—later on bourgeois—milieu in which the family lived. For several generations, it had lived up to its obligation to accomplish more and more and to gain more and more respect. The son was also supposed to continue this pattern, but he broke out of the family tradition. There were various psychological, social-psychological, and sociological reasons. Analysis showed that the son was repudiating his father's ideas in the sense of an antiauthoritarian revolt. He acted as one would expect in the case of an Oedipal problem: He fought his powerful father and his standards of achievement. His reaction was not just a passive retreat, which, according to psychoanalysis, would point to an oral problem. There is something essential in addition to all of this. The mother's family concept "What will people say?" contains an orientating side view to a social relational group. The father, with his emphasis on accomplishment, was deficient when it came to social contact. The son, on the other hand, placed more value on his mother's concept of being directly affirmed by other people. These other people were his peers, and their recognition was important to him. They enabled him to delineate himself opposite his father without continuing the tendencies of his family to keep rising in rank. This tendency had indeed become like an unstoppable landslide. The son thus abandoned the achievement principle that the preceding generations had submitted to and freed himself from it. In its place there was contact with other people, an ability to make friends that his parents had interpreted as just another indication of his degeneracy.

The family therapy took a different course than the parents had expected. The therapist did not deal solely with the so-called "sick person" but with the concepts of all the family members and the development of those concepts.

The son's symptoms were not a psychiatric syndrome, but a reaction to transmitted family concepts that had meant excessive expectations placed on the son. In the way he chose to avert this problem, he touched upon a weak point in the family: interpersonal relationships and social contact. In the case of his father, social contact had only been a means of achieving goals in his business. The mother was limited in her contacts in that she submitted to everything that other people said; her desire to assure her prestige and her reputation caused her to become more and more entrapped in rigid role playing. The more she

A Concept Family Tree

Ancestors (Collective Past) Ancestors

Great-grandfather:
"Be loyal and honest, but show what you can do" (achievement, honesty, thrift).

Great-grandmother:
"Treat us the way you do fine people" (achievement, justice, politeness, thrift).

Grandfather:
Favorite saying, "What you earn from your ancestors, make it your own so you really own it" (tradition, achievement, thrift).

Grandmother:
"Show everyone that you are something special; what will people say?" (industry/ achievement, politeness).

Father:
"If you can do something, you are someone. I have to be a success and have to work for it" (industry/achievement, time).

Mother:
"We've gotten somewhere. We're better and have to act accordingly" (politeness, achievement).

Son

(carrier of symptoms)

Relational group: The need to achieve is bourgeois repression.

Son's Concepts

"I don't just want to work; I also want to live."
"I want to live my own life. I could care less what people say."
"I'll dress the way I want."
"I like to be with people who have ideas like mine and not like my parents'."

needed other people for her image of herself, the more anxious she was about being seen differently than in the role she played under the direction of the game rules in her family (politeness). The son resolved this conflict by trying to free himself from the family's rules of courtesy, as in the saying "Once you've lost your reputation, there's not much left." But this did not all take place without a hitch. Instead of a career with a lot of chance of success, the boy dreamed of something artistic (fantasy as opposed to achievement). His process of detaching himself from his parents, as stormy as it appeared on the outside, was, inwardly, a slower process. His desire for dependence and security, which was partly unconscious, and his close ties to his mother led him to look for security in alcohol and other drugs. Alcoholism was the remnant of a family dependency that ran through several generations.

This differentiation of the concept family tree led to a differentiation of the family situation. The family's problem, which had simply been attributed to the son as the black sheep, was recognized as a problem for the entire family as it had existed in various forms over several generations.

We have found that the concept family tree has proved valuable in therapy for several generations, as set forth by Mendell and Fischer (1956), Sperling (1976), and Stierlin (1975). In this multi- and intergeneration therapy, grandparents and sometimes even the great-grandparents are included in the therapy along with the parents and children.

12. Tradition of Symptoms

The relationship of man to his environment is not static. It is dynamic and therefore always changing. His interaction with the environment changes it, and those changes have reactive effects on him. If patterns of thinking, feeling, and acting—man's culture—are not modified to reflect a constructive accommodation to those changes, the culture may easily become nonprogressive, eventually maladaptive, and ultimately genocidal.

—Daniel C. Jordan

Symptoms as well as concepts can be transmitted. In the relationships between the generations, they have their own continuity. They are transmitted and then reworked in the family situation. These symptoms are themselves expression of concepts regarding the body, the illness, and interpersonal communication. It is worthwhile to study the family history in terms of illnesses and symptoms. This does not take place just to trace the inheritance of certain illnesses. More important, it is essential to understand the meaning of the symptoms and the concepts behind them. They stand in close connection with the forms for dealing with conflict, the model dimensions, and the actual capabilities.

Psychosomatic illnesses are precisely the ones that frequently point to a family tradition, partly with a shift of symptoms within the generations. In this connection, we observed occurrences of asthma, migraine headaches, stomach problems, colon trouble, and functional heart ailments and "heart neuroses."

The latter are often found in conjunction with heart attacks and phobic reactions on the part of the parents. Other illnesses, which are considered to be primarily somatic, are not passed on directly. In this case, there are risk factors underlying the tradition, such as smoking, drinking, certain eating habits, tendency toward stress, et cetera. The symptom tradition is particularly revealing in the case of illnesses that one today labels as "endogenous." Parents of schizophrenics, for instance, are often deficient in social contact, very matter-of-fact, extremely punctual, neat, and ambitious and find it difficult to maintain a stable emotional relationship. These characteristics, which are designated as schizothymic or schizoid, affect the family atmosphere in a lasting way. The concepts underlying them are adopted by later patients in an even more severe form and express themselves in this clarity as the illness formation of schizophrenia. The tradition of the symptoms does not always occur so linearly, however, but develops out of a particular family tradition in which a number of symptom possibilities come into contact.

QUESTIONS ABOUT THE SYMPTOM TRADITION

1. Where were you treated previously? What symptoms and illnesses were treated? What explanations were given for these illnesses?
2. Which forms for dealing with conflict do you prefer? Which forms were preferred by your parents, your grandparents, et cetera? Which illnesses occur in your family, with your parents, grandparents, and other relatives? How were these illnesses handled? Which situations come to mind now?

Fewer material goods are passed on from one generation to the next than strategies for dealing with conflict and symptom formation, world views, and relational structures, transmitted from parents to children and then adopted by the latter and subsequently passed on again to their own children.

Epilogue

We can have both heaven and hell in this world.

An important feature of the model for Positive Family Therapy is that education and self-help are integral parts of the psychotherapy itself. Psychotherapy as reeducation refers directly to what was formed and learned in the upbringing. Through self-help the patient is encouraged as an active partner; he isn't merely the one who has to endure something. Self-help is a method of prevention and psychohygiene. It is an essential element in the psychotherapeutic process.

As forms of self-help, internal medicine offers such aids as fitness training, diet guidelines, and charts for keeping track of progress. Under the direction of a physician, the patient learns to actively do something to improve his health. In a similar way, educational problems, career conflicts, and marital difficulties can be approached by way of self-help.

For this reason I adopted the goal of writing a book that one could give to patients and clients within the framework of a medical and psychological practice as well in connection with consultation for specific problems. This book, as I envisioned it, should be useful as an aid in the therapeutic situation or the consultation process. The book was thus not conceived for specialists, but for a wide range of readers: students, young people, parents, business people, teachers, and educators as well as physicians and therapists.

Conflicts grow in the course of a person's development in confrontation with his environment; they are not unavoidable acts of fate. They are tasks and problems that we must try to solve.

The aspects of Positive Family Therapy promote a sense of self-worth, obviate the need for expressing hostility, and guarantee a compassionate social conscience—all prerequisites for world unity and peace.

THE GOLDEN TENT SPIKES

A dervish, whose joy was self-denial and whose hope was paradise, once met a prince, whose wealth exceeded everything the dervish had ever seen. The nobleman's tent, pitched outside the city for recreation, was made of precious fabrics, and even the spikes that held it up were solid gold. The dervish, who was used to preaching asceticism, attacked the prince with a flood of words about the futility of earthly wealth, the vanity of the golden tent spikes, and the fruitlessness of human endeavor. How eternal and majestic, on the other hand, were the holy places. Resignation, he said, was the greatest happiness. The prince listened seriously and with great thought. He took the dervish's hand and said, "For me, your words are like the fire of the midday sun and the clarity of the evening breeze. Friend, come with me, accompany me on the way to the holy places." Without looking back, without taking money or a servant, the prince set out on the way.

Astonished, the dervish hurried along behind him. "Lord," he cried, "tell me. Are you really serious about making a pilgrimage to the holy places? If you are, wait for me so I can go get my pilgrim's cloak."

Smiling kindly, the prince answered, "I left behind my wealth, my horses, my gold, my tent, my servants, and everything I owned. Do you have to go back just because of your cloak?"

"Lord," replied the dervish with surprise, "please explain to me—how you could leave all your treasures behind and even go without your princely cloak?"

The prince spoke slowly but with a steady voice. "I sank the golden tent spikes into the earth, but not into my heart."

Reviews of The Family as Therapist: New Strategies for Positive Family Therapy

"This book unites orient and occident, giving the reader a comprehensive view of healthy and pathological psychic life and behaviour. . . . This book does not only address those who professionally are entrusted with a psychotherapeutic task. It will be a rich source of psychological and pedagogic experiences also for those who—they may be parents or pedagogues—are engaged in pedagogic tasks."

Dr. Raymond Battegay
Psychiatric Policlinic
University of Basel

". . . found that the book is pedagogically strongly motivated and gives a great value to the possibilities of pedagogic influence with the object of developing more and more humanity. . . . I am convinced that amongst the abundant material of case histories many persons will find their own problem and ways to solve it."

Dr. M. Broglie
Medical superintendent

". . . With its fluent style which can be understood also by laymen, one would wish to recommend the book also to the physician—for his patient's sake and—who knows?—maybe for his own. . . ."

Erich Kocian
Medical journalist

". . . There is a convincing encouragement in guiding to planned changes in behaviour and in the basic belief of the author that people have variable possibilities and these certainly have influence on the patient. . . . The cases shown by the author represent an important clientele of a psychotherapeutic practice—patients for whom the practitioner frequently has no help. The reader will therefore find valuable suggestions and popular guidelines for actual help in his way of living."

Dr. Lilo Süllwold
Psychiatric Center
University Clinic
Frankfurt/Main

". . . In a short therapy which is concentrated upon the conflict, the individual patients, the partners or family groups are made independent as fast as possible by systematic self-analysis or a joint, clarifying discussion."

Dr. Wolfgang Kretschmer
Research Institute for Medical Psychology
and Constitutional Biology, Tübingen

". . . This book, which is of great use to a recovery of our present social and educational structure, should above all be taken up in the libraries of sanatoriums, rehabilitation centers and mothers' recovery homes as well as in the advisory boards for matrimony and education. . . ."

Dr. Eugen Schmidt,
Former manager of the Country Commission
for General Health Education

". . . My forensic practice has given me during the time a number of reserves regarding the human science of today. I therefore took [this] book up with a sceptical mind and was surprised that it kept me interested from beginning to end. I wish to pay [the author] the compliment that [he] did find a way of making many problems regarding interhuman relations clear also to the laymen and in a very attractive way, too. . . ."

Dr. Udo Schaefer
Attorney-General,
Heidelberg

". . . I support the concept of Positive Family Therapy by Dr. Peseschkian from West Germany. As an academician I found the approach proposed by Dr. Peseschkian to be extremely helpful. I am sure, that this book will be as successful as Dr. Peseschkian's previous publications."

Javad H. Kashani, M.D.
Director of Child and Adolescent Services
Mid-Missouri Mental Health Center

Bibliography

Abdu'l Baha. *Der Geheimnis göttlicher Kultur*. Frankfurt/Main, 1973.

———. *Paris Talks*. London: Baha'i Publishing Trust, 1951.

———. *Some Answered Questions*. Wilmette, Ill.: Baha'i Publishing Trust, 1981.

Adler, A. "Individualpsychologische Behandlung der Neurosen." In A. Adler, *Praxis und Theorie der Individualpsychologie* (Munich: Bergmann, 1920).

Alexander, F. *Psychosomatische Medizin: Grundlagen und Anwendungsgebiete*. Berlin and New York: Verlg de Gruyter, 1971.

Baha'u'llah. *Gleanings from the Writings of Baha'u'llah*. Wilmette, Ill.: Baha'i Publishing Trust, 1971.

Bales, R. F. "A set of Categories for the Analysis of Small Group Interaction." *American Social Review 15*, (1950), 146–159.

Battegay, R. "Narzissmus in seiner physiologischen und psychopathologischen Dimension," *Zeitschrift für Positive Psychotherapie 1* (1979).

Benedetti, G. "Die umweltbedingten Depression," *Zeitschrift für Positive Psychotherapie 6* (1984).

Bernstein, B. "Aspects of Language and Learning in the Genesis of the Social Process, *The Journal of Child Psychology and Psychiatry* (1961), 313–24.

Bernstein, B. "Language and social class" in: The British Journal of Sociology, 11, 217–276, 1960.

Boszormenyi-Nagy, J., and G. Spark. *Invisible Loyalties*. New York, 1973.

Bray, G. A. "Jejunoileal Bypass, Jaw Wiring, and Vagotomy for Massive Obesity." In A.J. Stunkard (Ed.), *Obesity*, (Philadelphia: W. B. Saunders, 1980), 369.

Brown, R. A. "Memories of Abdu'l Baha. Recollections of the early days of the Baha'i Faith in California" Baha'i Publishing Trust, Wilmette, Ill. 1980.

Dreikurs, R., and E. Blumenthal. *Eltern und Kinder, Freunde oder Feinde*. Stuttgart, 1973.
Erikson, E. H. *Childhood and Society*. New York: Norton, 1950.
Esslemont, J. E. *Baha'u'llah and the New Era*. New Delhi: The Baha'i Publishing Trust, 1978.
Frankl, V. E. *Der Wille zum Sinn: Ausgewählte Vorträge über Logotherapie*. Bern: Verlag Hans Huber, 1972.
Freud, Anna. *Das Ich und die Abwehrmechanismen*. London: Imago, 1946.
Freud, S. *Das Ich und das Es*. In *Complete Works*, Vol. 13 (Frankfurt/Main: S. Fischer Verlag, 1963).
———. *Neue Folge der Vorlesungen zur Einführung in die Psychoanalyse*. In *Complete Works*, Vol. 15 (London: Imago, 1940).
Gordnon, T. *Familienkonferenz, die Lösung von Konflikten zwischen Eltern und Kind*. Hamburg, 1972.
Grossman, S. P. "Role of the Hypothalamus in the Regulation of Food and Water Intake," *Psychol. Rev. 82*, (1975), 200.
Hofstätter, P. R. *Einführung in die Sozialpsychologie*. Stuttgart, 1973.
Innerhofer, P. "Ein Regelmodell zur Analyse und Intervention in Familie und Schule," *Zeitschrift Klin. Psychol. 3* (1974), 30–45.
Jackson, D. D. "Family interaction, family homeostasis and some implications for conjoint family therapy," *Psychiatry Quarterly 31*, (1957).
Jordan, D. C. "Durchbruch zur Selbstverwirklichung." In *Baha'i Briefe 37* (1969).
Jung, C. G. *Psychologische Typen*. In *Complete Works*, Vol. 6 (Rascher, 1960).
Klein, M. *The Psychoanalysis of Children*. London: Hogarth, 1932.
Kohut, H. *Restoration of the Self*. New York: International Universities Press, Inc., 1977.
Levi-Strauss, C. "The Family." In H. L. Shapiro, *Man, Culture and Society* (New York, 1956).
Luban-Plozza, B., and W. Pöldinger. *Der psychosoamtisch Kranke in der Praxis*. Munich: Lehmanns, 1971.
Mendell, D., and S. Fischer. "An Approach to Neurotic Behavior in Terms of a Three-Generation Family Model." In *Journal of Nervous and Mental Disease 123*, (1956) 171–180.
Meng, H. *Psychohygieneische Vorlesungen*. Basel, 1958.
Minuchin, S., and A. Barcai. "Therapeutisch induzierte Familienkrise." In Sager and Kaplan, *Handbuch der Ehe-Familien-, und Gruppentherapie*, Vol. 2 (Munich, 1973) 389–97.

Mitscherlich, A. *Krankheit als Konflikt: Studien zur psychomatischen Medizin II*. Frankfurt/Main: A. Aufl. Suhrkamp, 1968.
Niemöller, M. "Vortrag an der Weltkonstituante 1968 Interlaken." In *Baha'i Briefe, 35* (1969), 907–13.
Nietzsche, F. *Also sprach Zarathustra*. Leipzig, Alfred Kröner.
Peseschkian, N. *Auf der Suche nach Sinn: Psychotherapie der kleinen Schritte*. Fischer Taschenbuch, 1983.
———. "Les cinq phases de la Psychotheŕapie positive." In *Hexagon Roche,* Vol. 12, No. 4 (1984).
———. "Positive Psychotherapy in Medical Practice." In *Hexagon Roche,* Vol. 10, No. 3 (1982).
———. *Positive Psychotherapie: Theorie und Praxis einer neuen Methode*. Frankfurt/Main: S. Fischer Verlag, 1977.
———. "Psychosocial Norms in Medical Practice—Minor Emotional Trauma." In *Hexagon Roche,* Vol. 11, No. 2 (1983).
———. *Psychotherapie des Alltagslebens: Training zu Partnerschaftserziehung und Selbsthilfe*. Fischer Taschenbuch, 1977.
———. *The Merchant and the Parrot: Mideastern Stories as Tools in Psychotherapy*. New York: Vangage Press, 1982.
Rosenman, R. H., R. J. Brand, R. I. Sholtz, and M. Friedman. "Multivariate Prediction of Coronary Heart Disease during 8.5 Year Follow-Up in the Western Collabarative Group Study." *American J. Cardiol. 37* (1976), 903–10.
Schaefer, Udo. *The Imperishable Dominion*. Oxford: Georg Ronald, 1983.
Scott, J. P. "Individual Aggression as a Cause of War." In R. D. Givens and M. A. Nettleship (Eds.), *Discussions on War and Human Aggression* (The Hague and Paris: Mouton Publishers, 1976).
Secord, P. F., and C. W. Backmann. *Social Psychology*. London, 1964.
Shakespeare, W. *Hamlet, Prince of Denmark*. In *The Complete works of William Shakespeare,* edited by W. J. Craig (London: Henry Pordes, 1977).
Shogi-Effendi. *Die Weltordnung Baha'u'llahs*. Baha'i Verlag, Frankfurt/Main: Baha'i Verlag, 1973.
Spark, G. M. "Grandparents and Intergenerational Family Therapy," *Family Process 13* (1974), 225–37.
Speck, R. V., and C. L. Attneave. "Die Intervention in grössere Sozialsysteme." In *Handbuch der Ehe-, Familien- und Gruppen-therapie,* Vol. 2 (Munich, 1973), 510–44.
Spitz, R. A. *Die Entstehung der ersten Objektbeziehungen*. Stuttgart: Klett, 1960.

Stekel, W. *Frigidity in Woman,* Vol. 1 and 2. New York: Liveright Publ. Corp., 1943.
Stierlin, H. *Von der Psychoanalyse zur Familientherapie.* Stuttgart, 1975.
Stokvis, B. *Kulturpsychologie und Psychohygiene.* Stuttgart, 1965.
Watzlawik, P., J. H. Beavin, and D. D. Jackson. *Menschliche Kommunikation, Formen, Störungen, Paradoxien.* Bern, 1969.
Winnicott, D. W. *Playing and Reality.* London: Tavistock Publications, 1971.

Index

GPSR Compliance

The European Union's (EU) General Product Safety Regulation (GPSR) is a set of rules that requires consumer products to be safe and our obligations to ensure this.

If you have any concerns about our products, you can contact us on ProductSafety@springernature.com

In case Publisher is established outside the EU, the EU authorized representative is:

Springer Nature Customer Service Center GmbH
Europaplatz 3
69115 Heidelberg, Germany

Batch number: 10844627

Printed by Printforce, the Netherlands